Habits of Seven Highly Successful Juicers

Shane Whaley and Angela Von Buelow

Copyright ©2014 Shane Whaley and Angela Von Buelow

All rights reserved. This book may not be reproduced in any form, in whole or in part (beyond the copying permitted by US Copyright Law, Section 107, "fair use" in teaching or research, Section 108, certain library copying, or in published media by reviewers in limited excerpts), without written permission from the author.

The views expressed in this book should not be taken as expert instruction or commands. The reader is responsible for his or her own actions. The authors do not assume any responsibility or liability whatsoever on the behalf of the purchaser or reader of these materials.

At times, links might be used to illustrate a point, technique, or best practice. These will reference products we have found useful, but please do your own research, make appropriate comparisons, and form your own decisions as to which product will work best for you. Links to our website or products are used for illustration, because we are familiar with these examples.

The information, ideas, and techniques in this book are not medical advice or treatment, but rather knowledge intended to assist the reader. It is the responsibility of the reader to seek treatment for any medical, mental, or emotional conditions that might warrant professional care.

Please note: some links included in this book will generate a commission for Juicing Radio, should you decide to purchase an item. All products have personally been tried and tested by Shane and Angie. We only recommend books and movies that have helped us with our own success. Links might be used to illustrate a point, technique, or best practice. These will reference products that we have found useful, but please do your own research, make appropriate comparisons, and form your own decisions as to which products will work best for you.

ISBN: 1503206963

ISBN-13: 978-1503206960

Dedication

Angie and Shane dedicate this book to Joe Cross (*Fat, Sick and Nearly Dead*) for all his hard work in bringing juicing into the mainstream.

We will always be very grateful to Joe and other juicing pioneers who have changed our lives, and the lives of many others, for good!

Shane and Angie would also like to dedicate this book to Cliff Ravenscraft—The Podcast Answer Man, www.podcastanswerman.com—without whom Juicing Radio would still be a dream and not a weekly reality.

This book is dedicated to our Juicing Radio listeners. Each one of you gives us the energy and motivation to keep delivering to you inspiring podcast content every week. Thank you!

Contents

Foreword iii

Introduction... 1

Chapter 1 Tanya
    Chooses Juicing over Gastric Bypass... 9

Chapter 2 Ben
    Changes His Lifestyle to Be Active with His Family............... 25

Chapter 3 Leslie
    Chooses Positive Results... 41

Chapter 4 Angie
    Shares Visions of Success 59

Chapter 5 Brian
    Determined to Make a Change... 77

Chapter 6 Nancy
    Transforms Her Life to a Wholeness Perspective 91

Chapter 7 Shawny
    Affirms Her Process to Health 107

Shane's 7 Keys to Successful Juicing Weight Loss............................. 129

Joe Cross Talks about his Health Journey and
    How He's Not Perfect... 155

Resources.. 201

About the Authors... 205

Connect with Social Media.. 207

Foreword

I never would've thought that at my age I'd be writing about friends I made at summer camp. However, I became friends with Shane and Angie at Camp Reboot. Stacy, my wife who is a registered dietitian, was interviewed in the Joe Cross documentary, *Fat, Sick and Nearly Dead.* Part of her work is to find combinations of juiced fruits and vegetables that are helpful for treatments and also taste delicious.

Stacy and I have a private practice, Wellness Guides (www.wellnessguides.org), where we help clients achieve and maintain a healthy weight. We believe that nutrition and psychology go hand-in-hand when it comes to wellness and weight management.

Joe Cross asked me to participate in Camp Reboot as a lecturer on behavioral psychology, motivation, and mindfulness. I was blessed with the task of interviewing the successful rebooters about their journeys of wellness, hoping to highlight the psychological factors during a reboot. Joe thought that these success stories would be motivating for any beginning juicers, and my goal was to highlight changes in each person's motivation that led to improved health and wellness behaviors.

Shane volunteered to go first. Spend any time with him and you'll experience his verve for living healthy. His story was one many people could relate to: "How did I get here story?" It's a common theme as people often explain that their weight gain was so gradual. One day they were 50 pounds overweight. With busy lives and constantly changing schedules, eating became something to try to "fit in" to their schedules, rather than building the schedules around.

Shane's a good, hard-working man, who let his diet and exercise lapse. He worked hard to regain control of his health and change the trajectory of his life. He attributes his successful weight loss to juicing, but I think that his tenacious attitude and willingness to connect were also major values. Shane was more connected to his career, and his health was not primary. It took a reconnection with "who he wanted to be" to initiate this journey. This reconnection is difficult, but Shane did it!

As I listened, I was touched by the heroic wellness journeys these wonderful people had traveled, and also by their intense joy in sharing it. Each shared their stories eloquently, and they all shared the belief that if they could do it, so can you. Each story detailed the importance of healthy changes, and how juicing was a major factor in improving their confidence that it could be done. One other aspect was clear during the stories: it was a CONNECTION with the juicing community that made all the difference.

Shane and Angie invited me to be a guest on Juicing Radio, so Angie and I spent time on the phone discussing the segment. Angie's earlier career had educated her quite well about food, but not so much about maintaining wellness in her life. For her, things were a bit more complex, and her journey of wellness is another common theme: "It's not what I'm eating, as much as it's what's eating at me." People often use the term "emotional eating," however; I believe they are talking about "eating as coping." Coping is complex and leads to a different wellness journey for people who eat to cope.

As a food writer, Angie knew about high quality, taste, and presentation. She knew that the food we eat was more than just sustenance for the body; it was essential to being human. We talked about the role of food in our relationships and that time shared with others is often based around food. Angie understood this concept, which helped with her successful journey to a healthier lifestyle.

When Shane and Angie asked me to write a foreword for this book, I was more than glad to share my thoughts. The personal stories of successful juicers that you read are inspiring and motivating. Motivation is a huge part of staying healthy. Most people *know* what to do to be healthy, however, healthy behavioral change is not about learning information, but rather it's about maintaining motivation.

This book, *Habits of Seven Highly Successful Juicers,* and the weekly podcasts on Juicing Radio are excellent resources to help educate and motivate you to begin your successful journey to weight loss and a healthier lifestyle!

Dr. Russell Kennedy
Wellness Guides
October 2014

Introduction

"If it's to be, it's up to me."
—Brian Tracy

Have you ever wanted to lose 20 pounds, 40 pounds, 60 pounds (or more), while also safely and dramatically improving your health, energy, mental clarity, motivation, and even your career? Then this could be one of the most important books you will ever read.

Why You Might Want to Listen to Us

As the hosts of "Juicing Radio—The Juicing Podcast," we, Shane and Angela, can back that up with our own testimonies.

Shane went from being an overweight sales rep to an energetic, vibrant vice president of sales with his first juice fast in 2010. Shane lost 80 pounds, earned a senior promotion, and now runs half marathons.

Angie saw Shane's change in health and it inspired her to start juicing. She also started exercising, dropped 86 pounds, and went on to run several half marathons! She secured a major career promotion and has been featured in a *Woman's World*

Magazine focus on juicing. She has also appeared in Joe Cross's *Reboot with Joe* book and was a guest on *The Dr. Oz Show*.

You might be wondering why you would want to follow our suggestions. We are not juicing celebrities or gurus; we are two ordinary people who achieved phenomenal success through repeated juice fasts, consistent juicing, cleaner eating, and moderate exercise. We want to share how that happened.

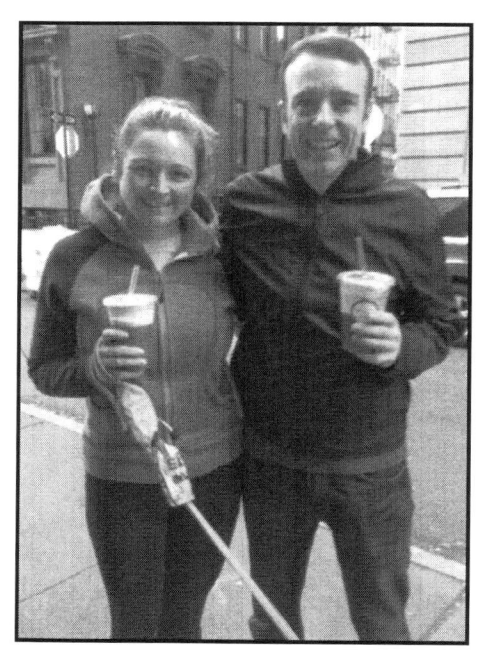

What Happened after Our Success with Juicing

Following our juicing success, we started a blog, "RunningOnJuice.com," and we communicated with thousands of people who had tried a juice fast but failed.

Most of them had the recipes and the juicer but lacked a vital ingredient, what we call "mental juice." What we put into our minds is just as important as the produce we put into our juicers and/or blenders.

Our mission has always been to support people through the juicing process. So we started the world's first weekly juicing podcast to deliver a glass of mental juice twice a week.

The podcast—Juicing Radio (www.juicingradio.com)—is now downloaded more than 30,000 times every month. We interview juicing success stories, and while we speak to some of the legends of juicing, most of our conversations are with ordinary folks, from different backgrounds, lifestyles, ages, and races, who wanted to change their lives for good.

How This Book Came to Be

In 2014, we decided to focus on seven successful juicers who have achieved phenomenal success. In this series, "The Habits of 7 Highly Successful Juicers," we honed in on their habits, their tips, and their tricks that sustained them through their first juice fast or reboot. The series became wildly popular and many of our listeners asked us to publish the interviews in book form so they could read and review the information when they need inspiration as part of their juice fast and lifestyle changes.

The result of those requests is what you are holding in your hands. We have reproduced these inspiring interviews so you can read them when you need a mental boost, so you won't feel like giving up. Or you can read one interview every morning as you enjoy your first green juice to power you through the book.

What to Expect

Seven juicers, two men and five women, share their personal stories with you about why they wanted to start juicing, how they managed their first juice fast, and the compelling reasons they had to make their lives better. Some of these reasons include the following themes:

Better Health—avoid gastric bypass surgery, avoid knee surgery, increase stamina, avoid depression, lower blood pressure, alleviate disease symptoms, adds a wholeness perspective

Build Self-Confidence—increase self-esteem, try new adventures, increased mental outlook, interaction and networking with others, failure is not an option, life transforming

Increased Exercise—walking, running, swimming, start where you are with small steps

Enjoy Life More—get out in nature, interact with children/grandchildren, no more sluggish lifestyle, happier

A Gift to Yourself—this is the most loving gift that you can give yourself; it becomes a spiritual, mental, physical, and emotional way of living.

Two Bonus Chapters

Shane shares his personal seven keys to juicing success. He gives you seven strategies that helped him drop 80 pounds and change his life for good. In addition, there is a chapter of a podcast with *Fat, Sick and Nearly Dead* movie maker and "Rebooter in Chief" Joe Cross, who is mentioned in every interview as one of the primary reasons that juicers wanted to begin the process to lose weight and improve their health through a juice fast.

We Are Here to Help

We know how difficult it can be to change poor lifestyle habits to positive choices that will enhance your physical, mental, and emotional well-being. We are here to help you! The successful juicers you meet in this book give you personal stories, insightful suggestions, and an incredible foundation to know that you will succeed in your goals!

We invite you to read these astounding stories, and we welcome you to begin your journey with us. It's an adventure that will give you a better outlook on life, a healthier physical body for life, and greater confidence to meet your specific life goals.

What are you waiting for? Start your transformation now! Paraphrasing Brian Tracy's quote: *"If it's to be, it's up to you."*

Get your free copy of
How to Get Started with Juicing
and receive free email juice coaching (but not spam—that's not healthy).

Sign up at www.juicinghabits.com.

JUICING RADIO

Shane and Angie interview a juicing success story every week on Juicing Radio.

Sign up for updates and never miss an episode at

JuicingRadio.com

Awesome! by txlonghorn03

Even as someone who is in the health industry and whose life was changed by juicing, I really thought a podcast on juicing could get stale fairly quick. I was very wrong! Shane and Angie do a great job keeping things fresh and inspiring. Give this a listen. No gimmicks or trends here. This is what juicing is all about.

Chapter 1
Tanya
Chooses Juicing over Gastric Bypass

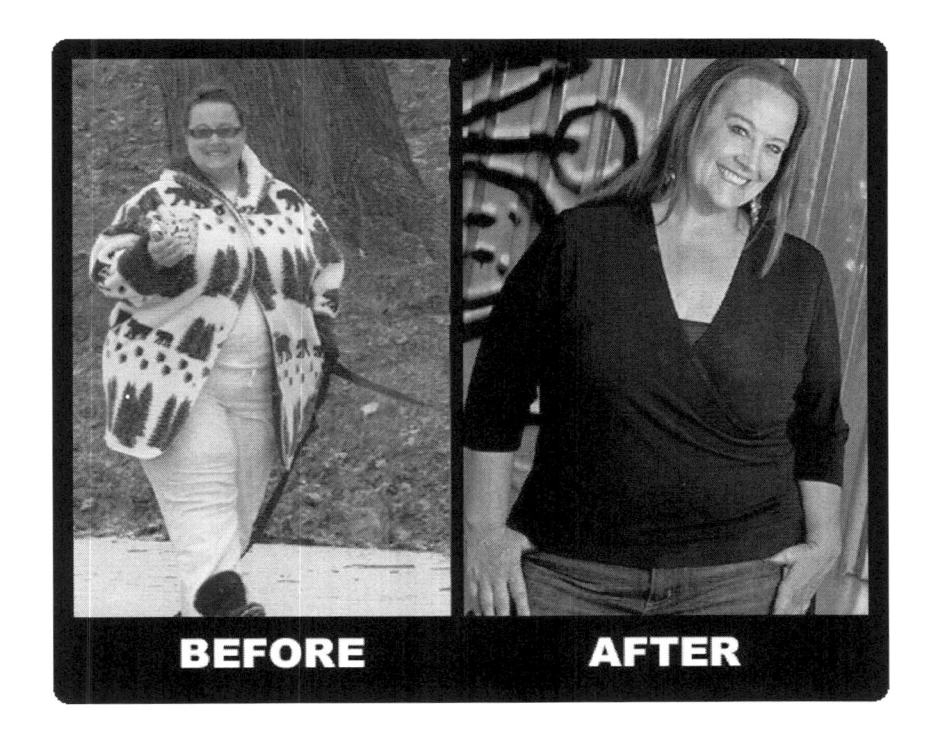

BEFORE **AFTER**

Shane: Hi, we have Tanya on the line. Tanya, whereabouts are you from?

Tanya: Hi, Shane. I'm from Queens, New York.

Shane: You're not far from me. How much have you lost, weight-wise, since you did your very first reboot?

Tanya: Actually, right now, because I weighed myself this morning, I'm down 96 pounds.

Shane: 96 pounds, that is incredible! So for those of you who are tuning in and you are doing your first reboot, cleanse, juice fast, juice feast, whatever you want to call it, you really need to be inspired by Tanya and the fact that she's lost 96 pounds through juicing.

If I could take you back to the very start, what made you start a juicing detox?

Tanya: Actually, it was sparked from my doctor suggesting that I have gastric bypass surgery, so I could alleviate the pain that I was feeling from a knee injury. She suggested, as a way to lessen that pain and to lose weight, to go for gastric bypass surgery. That really wasn't something that I was interested in pursuing, you know, having surgery.

Shane: Wow, so it was the thought of going for the operation that prompted you to say, "Okay, I'm going to try to do a detoxing program"?

Tanya: Yes.

Shane: Which detox juicing program did you follow?

Tanya: I actually saw Joe Cross's movie, *Fat, Sick and Nearly Dead,* so I started following a lot of information that I received off his website. There were a lot of recipes and I did some reading and that's really how I jumped in. After I saw his movie, I ordered my juicer and the minute it arrived, I started my juicing program right away.

Shane: Where was that in terms of the timeline? You had the news from your doctor that she wanted you to have the gastric bypass. Had you already seen Joe's movie at that stage or did that come later?

Tanya: No, that came later. I actually saw her in January, and we had talked about my weight issues at that time and I was just like, "Yeah, I know, I'm working on it." It wasn't until I went to the doctor in May, when my knee started bothering me, that she brought up the gastric bypass surgery. She put that seed in my mind and also recommended that I start physical therapy for the pain in my knee. My physical therapist was the one who recommended the movie, probably in June. It took about six weeks before I actually watched the movie in July. July 22 is when I originally started my first reboot.

Shane: I find it fascinating, Tanya, because there are a lot of people who I see who want to lose weight. I suggest that they watch *Fat, Sick and Nearly Dead.* A lot of them don't. It's almost as if they're too scared to be confronted with the truth. It's interesting to hear that it took you six weeks to watch the movie. I know people close to me who it took two or three months before they'd even watch it.

Tanya: Right, I think sometimes you go through life with these rose-colored glasses and you don't see what you actually look like. I always tend to look at myself from the nose up. I never really looked from the nose down. I guess I was too scared to look down. But you really need to look at the whole picture to see exactly where you are. It took watching that movie and my doctor suggesting a bypass—that's when I really took a good look at myself and knew I needed to make a change. I mean, I wasn't getting any younger.

Shane: Sure. Let's go back to the beginning. You've got your juicer and then you went to the Reboot with Joe website to follow Joe's reboot guidance?

Tanya: Yes. I got a lot of information from his website. I saw the movie. I bought my juicer, and then I just jumped right into juicing. On Joe's website it gives a little bit more of a guided way to start off with a reboot—a couple of tips about what you should do before to prepare your body—but I just jumped right in, I dove right in when I did it. Like I said, I saw the movie, I ordered my juicer, and I went out and bought a bunch of produce. Then I just started juicing away. Sometimes I juiced some stuff on my own, which didn't come out very well. Then I started following more of the recipes to at least get a feel for it, so I could know exactly what worked best with what, so it tasted good.

Shane: If you can remember the morning that you started, were you scared at all of telling yourself, "Wow, I'm going to try this juice-only thing." Did you have any fear?

Tanya: I don't know if it was so much fear as determination. I knew what I wanted to do. I didn't know how long I would do it, so I was just taking it one day at a time and making sure I could get through that first day. I think I was just more psyched for it than really scared. I just had my mindset that this was something that I wanted to do, and I was not going to let anything interfere with my goal.

Shane: I think you are a remarkable woman because I remember my first detox. That was before *Fat, Sick and Nearly Dead,* so I didn't have that really strong, positive frame of reference. I doubted it during the first five or six days whether this was healthy, whether it was a good thing for me. I think it's great that from day one you were resolute that this was going to be successful for you.

During that first week, did you watch any movies or read any books? Was there anything else that you looked to for inspiration in the early part of your juice cleanse?

Tanya: Just the Joe Cross site. And I found the *Juicing for Dummies* Facebook page and the Running on Juice website. I was looking for a lot of that information. I would do Internet searches and read some stuff. I'd really like to start reading more. There's a lot that I still need to learn now, so I'd like to start reading a little bit more. I've seen interesting items, so I've been writing down those I want to look into and read. That's all the places that I really looked to for inspiration when I was first starting out.

Shane: Why do you think your first juice cleanse was so successful, Tanya?

Tanya: I think it was because I had set my mind that I wanted to do it. I went through going to friends' bridal showers, and Halloween at work, where they brought in bagels and candy. I just sat there with my juice in hand.

Shane: I saw a photo of you the other day when everybody was eating pizza and you were there with your green juice. I did smile.

Tanya: Yes. That was me. They were all making fun of me.

Shane: Yeah, I know that well. During the early part of your cleanse, did you have an "aha" moment? When did things first click that you thought you knew, "This is right for me, this is going to work"?

Tanya: I think probably within the first two weeks, when I had dropped 20 pounds. I mean, I know a lot of that was water weight, but just the feeling of waking up without having a headache was great. Almost once a week I would get a migraine headache, so I'd be popping Advil. I still have not had a headache since I started juicing in July.

It's just the overall sensation of feeling good and feeling alive more than I ever have. Even within me, like my face, my eyes feel brighter, my skin looks better and it feels better. It's that general, over-all, well-being that you know you're doing positive things to your body and it's responding.

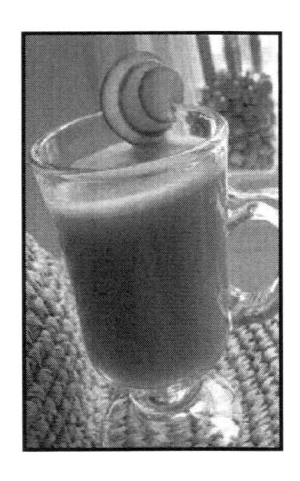

Shane: For those of you who might be on day two or day three of your reboot, your cleanse, really listen to what Tanya is saying. I know for me, day two and day three were the ones where I really struggled. My energy was the lowest, and I was really was kind of angry and moody and didn't feel good. It's about day four when suddenly you find an abundance of energy and you start to see and feel the benefits.

I don't know if it was the same for you, Tanya. The first couple of days were rough. Like Joe, in the movie, they're pretty rough. Then suddenly the benefits do come. Like when you said that within the first two weeks you dropped the weight and you weren't getting headaches.

For those of you who might be on day two, it might be hard to believe. You might be thinking, *This isn't right for me,* but *please* stick with it and push through it. Get to day four and day five and start to experience some the benefits that Tanya is discussing.

So, Tanya, what was the biggest challenge for you in the earliest days?

Tanya: The biggest challenge was just making sure that I was prepared for the next day. I juiced a lot at night to carry my stuff with me in my cooler bag the next day to work. Just making sure I was prepared and sometimes not buying too much produce because my refrigerator wasn't that big. I had a hard time keeping everything in my refrigerator.

Shane: During that time, the early part of the reboot, did you have any specific cravings and, if so, how did you work through overcoming those cravings?

Tanya: You know, I really didn't have too many cravings, other than walking into my apartment building and smelling all the things that people were cooking.

Shane: Yes.

Tanya: Near my apartment I actually have a juice bar, which, sad to say, I hadn't visited prior to juicing. But I have visited it a lot since I started.

Shane: I bet they loved you during your reboot.

Tanya: Yeah! I would just take in the smells and that kind of satisfied me. The only other craving I really had was for a mango salsa that I used to buy. What I did was take some of the ingredients that went into it and designed a juice around it, so that satisfied my craving.

Shane: Nice, that's interesting. Again, I think you're remarkable, Tanya, because most people in the early days of reboot are craving chocolate or cheeseburgers and instead you're craving mango salsa. On the big scale of things, that isn't bad, is it?

Tanya: No, not really.

Shane: I remember during my early detox, toward the end, I couldn't watch television. It was the same thing when I gave up smoking about ten years ago—you watch TV and you immediately notice how many people are smoking.

Tanya: I know.

Shane: With food, it was the same for me. I remember watching a James Bond movie, and I love James Bond, and I'm saying to myself, "I can't watch this, because he's eating a 15-course meal."

Tanya: I gave up smoking three years ago, too.

Shane: Congratulations, well done!

Tanya: Thanks, well you, too. Now, I can actually smell somebody smoking in the next car when I'm driving, which is so odd, because I could never smell it before. It's the same thing with the juicing. You notice what everybody's eating.

Shane: Everything!

Tanya: I was making fun of my coworkers yesterday because it was our holiday party and we had Chinese food, well, *they* had Chinese food. I told them, "Yeah, you guys will all be tired in about an hour, but I won't because I just had my juice."

Shane: Good for you. That's a great way of looking at it. That's a good mental strategy to cope with it.

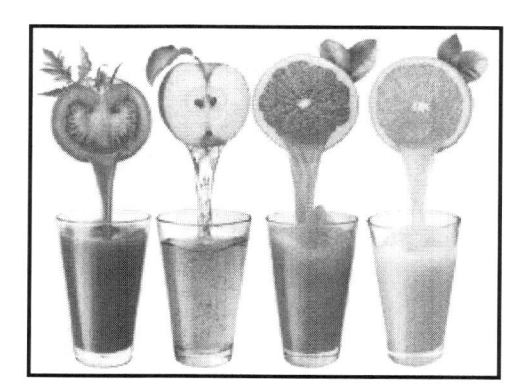

Tanya: Yes.

Shane: When you were on your detox, did you receive any negative feedback from friends and family?

Tanya: No, not really. Everybody was pretty much cheering me along, other than a couple of people at work saying, "Your food should be eaten, not drunk in a cup." My mother actually has been juicing in the morning for the past few weeks. My brother has tried it. My sister-in-law has tried it. I've kind of given some of them a little buzz to try to get involved with me and the whole juicing community. That's been a great support, and not really too many negative comments.

Shane: I think you're very fortunate to hear the positive, or not to get the negative. I think your transformation is absolutely amazing. I think of your family and your close friends who see the transformation that you've gone through, and also the fact that your knee isn't aching and you don't need a cane to walk. You look very fit from your photographs. I mean, I would be storming out of the house to go buy myself a juicer, if I were a friend of yours. That is such a validation that this process works.

Tanya: It does! It worked for me and it's still working for me. I'm still on my journey. I've still got a little ways to go, but it's great. I've never felt better in my life.

Shane: That's fantastic. What advice would you give to someone who wants to start a detox? What advice would give to someone who's never juiced before? What would you say to that person, Tanya?

Tanya: Just take it one day at a time. Don't put too much pressure on yourself. Just get through those first couple of days and really, after those first couple of days, it's downhill from there, because you start to reap the benefits of just giving your body all the nutrients that it needs, and it pays you back with favorable responses. You feel better, you start to look better. And it's a great feeling when you go to the doctor and there are positive results. My blood pressure's gone down and my blood work shows that everything's in tip-top shape.

Shane: Fantastic, congratulations! A little Twitter bird told me that your doctor had given you a good report.

Tanya: Yes, and I celebrated by buying myself a tandem skydive that I'll probably do sometime in the spring.

Shane: You're going to jump out of an aircraft?

Tanya: I did it ten years ago, so I figure I might as well do it again as a celebration for myself.

Shane: Celebration, okay. You're doing something very strange on New Year's Day, aren't you?

Tanya: I'm going to do the Polar Bear Plunge in Lake George. That's where you run into a nice, icy cold lake with a ton of other crazy people.

Shane: That is crazy. When I lived in Sweden, the guys would do that, but I always refused. I just couldn't jump into that cold. There's just no way.

Tanya: I've heard it's very invigorating, so if I'm starting this new year better than I was last year, I figure this is a good way to start it off.

Shane: Good for you. What habits did you create in the early part of your detox to help you succeed on your juice fast? You've already said that you would make the juices at night for the next day, which I think is a great habit to get into. Were there any other habits you can share with us that you brought into your new lifestyle?

Tanya: I learned to plan. I was never a planner before. I would always stop at the store on the way home from work and get my dinner. I never really cooked. Through juicing I've learned to really plan. For example, I plan for events. If I know I am going somewhere and there are going to be foods with lots of good smells, I make sure I have my juices and my water with me so that I have something to fall back on. I don't want to say, "Oh, my God, I'm so hungry." I want to try to stick to my juice fast, so I prepare myself for anything unexpected that could come up.

Shane: Good for you. They're great, solid habits that you've shared. Where can people follow your journey online? Like you said, you've got a bit more of a road to go, so people might want to see how you're doing.

Tanya: Actually, I'm writing for Juicefast.com. I just started a blog, so people can follow me there, or they can join me as a friend on my personal Facebook page: Tanya Hoffay.

Shane: How about your Twitter account? You use Twitter quite a lot, right?

Tanya: Yes. My Twitter is TEE468Y.

Shane: If you want to follow Tanya and keep an eye on her journey, I really suggest you do, especially if you're in the early stages of your reboot. If you're very lucky and you send Tanya an e-mail with a question, she might even answer you.

Tanya, your story is absolutely amazing. It's very inspiring. Thank you very much for sharing your journey and inspiring others!

Tanya: Thank you, Shane.

Tanya Hoffay Facebook Page

https://www.facebook.com/tanya.hoffay?fref=ts

Get your free copy of
How to Get Started with Juicing
and receive free email juice coaching (but not spam—that's not healthy).

Sign up at www.juicinghabits.com.

JUICING RADIO

Shane and Angie invite you to listen to a juicing success story every week on Juicing Radio.
Sign up for updates and never miss an episode at JuicingRadio.com.

New Juicer

by MinaFuji

I started listening to Juicing Radio the end of last year after I watched Joe's movie. Juicing Radio has given me lots of useful information and tips/tricks from experienced juicers! I listen to the podcasts over and over again. It seems like every time I listen to them, I learn something new! Shane and Angie, I thank you for all your hard work. I wanted to let you know how much I appreciate the both of you!

Chapter 2

Ben

Changes His Lifestyle to Be Active with His Family

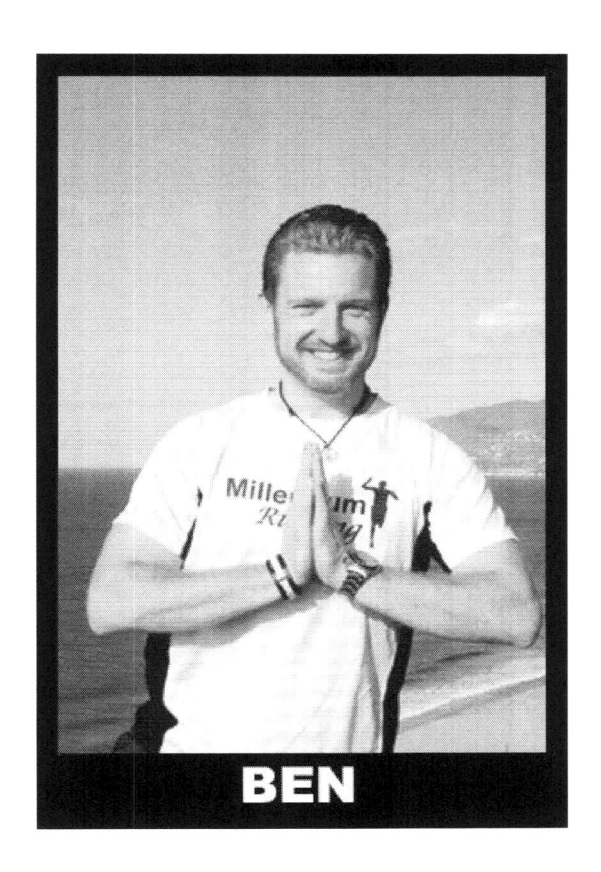

Shane: Welcome, Ben. How are you?

Ben: I'm great, Shane. How are you?

Shane: I'm wonderful. Which part of the country are you from?

Ben: I'm from Bedford, Massachusetts.

Shane: Massachusetts, great. Before we delve into other questions, how much weight did you lose through juicing?

Ben: Since September 2012, I've lost 115 pounds.

Shane: Wow, 115 pounds. That is amazing. That is incredible. We met at Camp Reboot and I know you had lost most of the weight by then. I can't even imagine what you looked like when you were 115 pounds heavier, Ben.

Ben: I can send you a picture if you really want to see it, but I don't like to show that off anymore.

Shane: I can imagine. I think the fact that you're one of our seven juicing success stories, people will understand that. But what was it that made you start a juice fast the very first time?

Ben: Well, a friend of mine sat me down and said, "If you don't change your life, you are going to die. And I am detrimentally worried about you, so just do something." He gave me some ideas of places to look and said, "I know you're not an avid reader, but there's a lot of stuff on Netflix." And over a couple of days, I just started to watch a bunch of health documentaries on Netflix.

The good thing about Netflix is once you've watched one, it gives you a recommendation: "Hey, watch this too." And the first one I watched was *Fat, Sick and Nearly Dead.* I was just really blown away by it. I saw how Joe Cross had amazing results in just 60 days. And I thought it looked fairly easy. It was something that I flashbacked to when I was a kid. I saw the Jack LaLanne commercials about 500 times. So I thought I'd go and get myself a juicer and I did.

Shane: Fantastic. Going through your journey now and having gone through it, your friend said to you "If you don't change your life, you're going to die." Is that something you would actually endorse now?

Ben: Yeah. At that point, now that I look back on it, even though I was still functioning—I still had a pulse and could walk around—I didn't have as much mobility as I do now. But in hindsight, I was already dead. I was just like a zombie. I had no real life to myself. I had no spirit, I didn't have anything.

I used to be so sedentary that I was just living on my couch, watching TV day in and day out, eating all day and just sleeping. So, I didn't really have anything of what life has to offer. Yes, I could have extended my life 10, 20 years maybe before a heart attack or something else got me. But for all intents and purposes, I was already dead at that point and I didn't want to keep going anymore.

Shane: I think we all relate to that. And I'm smiling here, Ben, because you've gone from this very sedentary lifestyle—like you said, you sat at home most of the day either sleeping, eating or on the sofa—and now, you're doing Spartan races, right?

Ben: Yes.

Shane: So, for those of us who don't know, what is a Spartan race?

Ben: A Spartan race is the pinnacle level of obstacle course racing. There are three different levels: a 3-plus mile race, a 7-ish mile race or a 13-ish mile race. It involves not only running, but you're running through woods, crawling through mud, jumping over fire, crawling underneath barbed wire, jumping over walls, and lifting heavy objects. It's an endurance race that challenges you through all levels of your body. And it also challenges you mentally.

Shane: Which program did you follow when you started juicing for the first time?

Ben: I didn't really follow any program. I went to the RebootWithJoe.com website, and I followed a few of the basic recipes. I tried to hold true to the theory that most of your juices should be 80 percent vegetable, 20 percent juice.

However, I like to follow the beat of my own drum. So, at first I followed a lot of the recommended recipes. But then, I just began to experiment with that 80/20 formula. I always found something that worked for me. If I created a juice that wasn't to my taste, I would try to sweeten it. You can really make a lot of juices sweeter—throw in some ginger, throw in some lemon or something like that—and that's basically what I did.

Shane: It's fascinating to hear that, because nearly everyone we've interviewed for this series has said the same thing. That when they began, there weren't a lot of recipes on Joe's site or they just started freestyle juicing where they were experimenting with all the different recipes. Most people have said exactly the same thing as you, Ben.

Ben: Yeah, that's really great. What I found is that you can really make any juice taste good. I researched the plant-based foods that had better nutritional value. Kale and spinach are the two hardcore juicing vegetables, but plain kale doesn't really do it for me. If you throw in a little bit of ginger, some apples or some carrots, you can make the juice taste like something that is very sweet and palatable.

Shane: During those early days of your juice fast, were you scared?

Ben: Yes, I was extremely scared. And I still get this reaction from people all the time. I just saw a very good documentary on a Facebook site called "Food, Inc" where someone posted that juicing is bad.

Shane: Oh, really?

Ben: Yeah. People still have all these negative predisposed opinions. Like they think that you're not going to get calories, they think that you're starving to death. They think it's just some weird trend.

So, that overwhelming negative attitude was the hardest thing for me to overcome. That was my biggest stumbling block, because I thought everyone was telling me I was crazy. But the thing I told myself was "I have nothing left to lose. And if this doesn't work, I'm still going to be in the same terrible position that I'm in, so what do I have left to lose?" And I did it and all of a sudden, I had these fantastic results. And now I let my own picture do the talking, you know?

Shane: I salute you. Because when I did my first juice fast in 2008, I gave up on day three. I mean, this was way before the movie, so I had no positive frame of reference. But everyone was telling me the same thing: I was crazy, it was insane. I gave up.

And then, it took me another 18 months before I completed my first seven-day juice fast. So, I commend you for staying strong and for not listening to friends and family who say negative stuff. It's very easy, certainly the first few days of a juice fast, to cave in and think, "Oh, yeah, everyone is telling me I'm going to get kidney stones" or "It's bad for me, I'll give up."

We've all been scared and had people say negative things to us. However, the successful juicers all pushed through and have achieved amazing results like you've heard already. "Ben has dropped 115 pounds and he's now running Spartan races." But these are not fake testimonials. These are ordinary people who have decided to juice and achieved remarkable results.

Ben, the question for you is this: "Why do you think your first reboot was so successful?"

Ben: I think I had the perseverance to stick through it. You're not always as perfect with it as you want to be, because perfection is something very hard to strive for. But basically, the biggest thing for me to remember was whenever you even slightly fall off the horse, you get back on. So, even if I did have a stumbling block, I would know that I would always have a juice there waiting for me.

I noticed after about the end of the first week, I started to get cravings for the juice. And I started to feel, within less than a week, all those positive effects right away. I used to be so sedentary, so drawn down, and I had no energy at all.

After about five days, all of a sudden, I was getting up on my own. I didn't have to press the "snooze" button 15 times, which, 115 pounds ago, was very difficult because I used to have very bad sleep apnea and didn't sleep well.

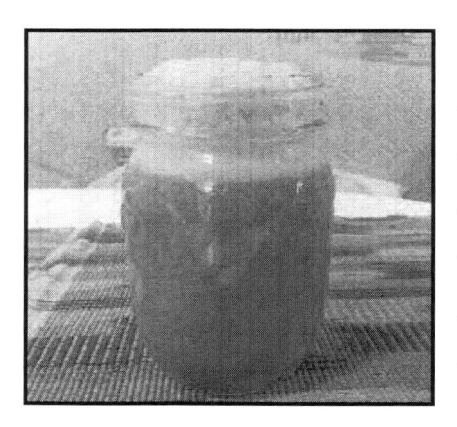

I just noticed all these positive effects right away and I kept that in my mindset. I knew that things would just keep building. And sure enough, they did. They continue to build today.

Shane: Absolutely, I hear you. What was the biggest challenge for you during that first week, in particular, or the early days of the juice fast?

Ben: Definitely, the biggest challenge, number one, was not being prepared. Because what I noticed is that you process the juice in your digestive system relatively quickly. So, once you drink a juice, within about two hours, three hours tops, you just start to feel hunger again right away. And if you don't have another juice prepared and ready, it really messes with you.

So, by the end of the first week, I found out how to store juice. And that's been my staple because I wouldn't have been able to have success if I hadn't done it this way. I made all my juices for the next day the night before, and I stored them in bottles, in Mason jars in the fridge, because juice will keep for up to three days.

If you try to make one juice at a time and go through the lengthy process of just making 500 milliliters or 1 liter, and then you have to clean out the juicer and rinse it again, it's a very tedious process. So, the biggest thing that helped me was just making it all in a "one-stop shop" the night before, and then I had a whole day's worth of juice. So, whenever I had those hunger feelings, I always had a juice ready for me.

Shane: Yeah, that's very smart advice. And again, that's something I'm hearing as a common thread—that people are preparing their juices in advance.

During your first week, Ben, did you have any specific cravings during your detox?

Ben: My biggest thing was coffee. The juice didn't actually become palatable and I didn't crave them for about five to seven days. So, in the first three days, they do taste kind of unnatural. And I was still trying to imagine that I'm drinking a heavy milkshake or this thing had some pizza in it or something. That's basically what I was telling myself to psych me up.

But what I noticed right away is the adaptability of the human body. Somewhere along the line, whenever it was, 10-plus years ago, I got adapted to processed food. And that's what I started to crave, that's what I lived off of. So, when you have a diet of processed foods, you're adapted to it. So, then, when you have something natural and clean and you eat it, it tastes unnatural to you. But the process is you can flip the coin.

So, now I'm adapted to drinking juice and eating clean food. And if I eat a slice of pizza, that's going to make me instantly sick, give me gas, and cause bloating. But the same thing happens the other way around. When you're normally used to just eating processed food and you have a juice, you get these weird cramps and gas. But it's just amazing how fast your body can work that out. It only takes about a week, I found, for me to adapt.

Shane: I absolutely agree with you on that. So, what advice would you give someone? Maybe it's day one of their juice fast and they're a little nervous, a little scared. They know they need to lose some weight. They know they need to change and turn their life around. What advice would you give to that person if you sat with them right now, Ben?

Ben: My biggest piece of advice would be to have mental preparation. So, when you are ready to start your first day, don't do it like I did. Don't make one juice at a time. Have your whole day prepared, and that prepares you mentally. I think that mental preparation is the most important key factor.

So, when you're preparing yourself the night before, you're also mentally rehearsing your next day. So, when you're making your juice, you're thinking, *This is what I'm going to have for breakfast, this is what I'm going to have for lunch. This is how I'm going to store it.* And you have all these positive thoughts going through your head of what tomorrow is going to be like and what the day after that is going to be like.

And then, you start to build yourself: "What's it going to be like in six months? What's it going to be like in a year?" And those positive affirmations, I think, are what helped me carry myself forward. I always had the knowledge to go through a preparation process. Every day, I gave myself positive affirmations and associated them with juicing.

Shane: Again, that's something I really support, Ben. And I think the majority of us who succeed on a juice fast, detox cleanse, reboot, call it what you will, do a lot of visualization to pump ourselves up. We drink what Angie and I call the "mental juice."

Because it's not just the green juice you put in your body, it's what you're putting into your mind. And it's very easy, it's like anything else. Giving up cigarettes or taking up exercise, it's very easy to beat yourself up and give up. You really need to strengthen your brain and your mind and your mindset to "Yeah, I'm doing this for A, B and C reasons. And in a month's time, I'm going to be able to get up and walk for half an hour around my neighborhood instead of getting in the car." In the beginning, you set smaller goals.

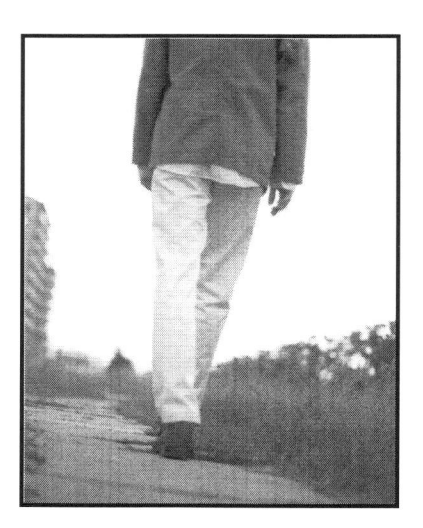

I'm fairly certain that on day one you didn't say to yourself "Yeah, man. I'm going to juice and I'm going to run a Spartan race."

Ben: No, in the beginning, I thought it was just a joke. My friend who encouraged me has been doing this for several years. I'd lost touch with him over the years, but we reconnected and he challenged me to change my life. I thought he was calling me out as a joke. I thought, *Yeah, I would never do that.* But at the same time, I just wanted to get my health back. I thought, *At least I want to be there for my kids. I want to see my grandkids someday, if I'm ever going to have any.*

And that was my immediate goal. I live close to a lake, but I couldn't even walk to it a year-and-a-half ago. I just wanted to walk down to the water without having to catch my breath 20 times. I wanted to walk there nonstop. That was the building block for the next step. The next step, after I made it to the shore, was to try to make it around the neighborhood. And then, within a month, I realized, *Wow, I'm actually getting a lot of results here. Maybe I can actually run someday.*

About six months went by and I went for my first run. It was only a few hundred meters of a sprint, but it was something. And once you have these little building blocks, they just keep building.

I met you in August, a week before I had done my first Spartan race. Now, I've done four races. My next one, I want to do at the elite level. So, yeah, you just keep building.

What I found with juicing is that your results are really exponential. People even say in the regular weight loss world, "You should strive for a pound a week," and I was kind of striving for that without doing a ton of extra effort. It just kind of happens.

What I've noticed with juicing, it just makes a lot of things happen in your body, not only physically, but also mentally. I used to have some problems with depression and other issues like that. And I don't know the whole brain chemistry thing; maybe the juice goes up there and affects the neurons, but I know I feel better.

Shane: Well you know, Ben, I'm pleased to hear that. And I'm very careful on Juicing Radio about making claims about health. But I tell you what. I've heard from several friends of mine who suffered with bipolar disease that juicing helped get them off their meds and reduced some of those horrible symptoms of bipolar and depression. Now, I'm not saying that juice is going to do that for everyone, but I'm hearing this more and more from people.

Ben: That's how I try to say it to them. Obviously, I'm not a doctor and neither are you, and, as with any medical issue, I just encourage people to be informed, do research on the Internet. Unless you have some sort of allergy, you don't have a lot to lose by just experimenting with it.

Shane: Well, Ben, you did have a lot to lose and you lost it—115 pounds. Everyone at Juicing Radio applauds you, congratulates you. Thank you very much for sharing a little bit about your habits and how you've been so successful.

Ben: You're welcome, Shane. It was great.

Get your free copy of
How to Get Started with Juicing
and receive free email juice coaching
(but not spam—that's not healthy).

Sign up at www.juicinghabits.com.

JUICING RADIO

Shane and Angie invite you to listen to a juicing success story every week on Juicing Radio.

Sign up for updates and never miss an episode at JuicingRadio.com.

Just What I Needed!

by Ohio Juicer

This is an amazing podcast. I start an episode before I begin juicing for the day and it gets me fired up and motivated to finish the day strong. Shane and Angie are awesome and the interviews are great.

Chapter 3
Leslie
Chooses Positive Results

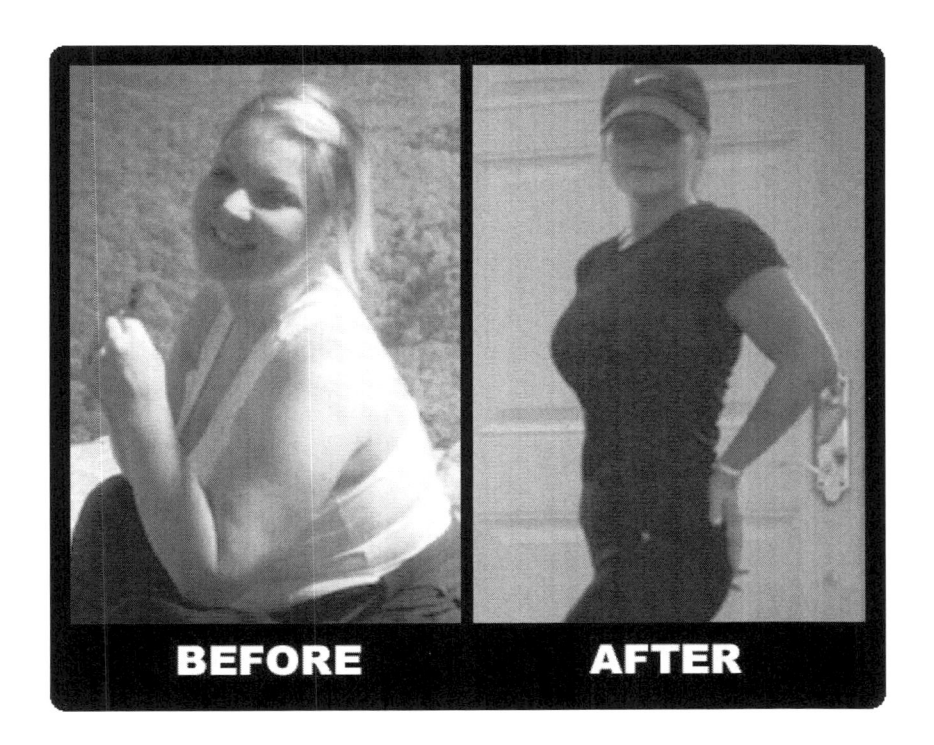

BEFORE **AFTER**

Shane: It's an immense pleasure to hear Leslie's experience. She lost 47 pounds by juicing and has really transformed her life. Juicing is now one of her major passions in life. Leslie set up the Juicing for Dummies Facebook Page and there are nearly 20,000 likes for the page. It is one of the busiest, most supportive online communities for juicing. Hi Leslie, please tell us about where in the world you are from?

Leslie: I am from the Nashville, Tennessee, area—a little town called Murfreesboro.

Shane: Can you explain to our listeners what made you start your very first juicing detox, or reboot, or cleanse?

Leslie: My first detox that I did, I decided to do after watching *Fat, Sick and Nearly Dead.* I had absolutely no doubt in my mind that I could do this, and I was ready for a challenge in my life. I was looking for change and this is the way that I found it.

Shane: Which program did you follow when you first did your reboot? Where did you get the information on recipes, or did you follow a plan or a program?

Leslie: Well, this is pretty easy, because at the time when I watched *Fat, Sick and Nearly Dead,* Reboot with Joe wasn't really up and going smoothly. It didn't have the plans like it does now, so I freestyled just like Mr. Joe did in *Fat, Sick and Nearly Dead.* That's pretty much all I did was follow what he did—drank the juice—for 30 days.

Shane: Wow, that's amazing that you did 30 days and freestyled it. So a lot of people, me included, really need a plan to get started. For example, my program has the five juices you need every day. Are there any tips that you can give to people who haven't freestyled, maybe because they're not online or don't have access to a plan?

Leslie: Well, as far as tips go, I'm not that different from other people, but I mostly pulled recipes out of my head. I suggest sticking to the main greens. Mr. Joe's recipe really covers everything. It fills you up. If you're just doing five to seven days, you don't need too much fruit because of the sugar that's in it. Stick mostly to main greens. That would be my biggest tip.

Shane: Were you scared during your first few days of doing this juice-only thing? Did you have any fear?

Leslie: No. I didn't. I think everybody might be a bit hesitant of the unknown. But failure, it just wasn't an option for me.

Shane: And why do you think your first reboot was so successful?

Leslie: My first detox was successful because I completed it. For the first time in my life, I set my mind to something and I accomplished it, and I saw amazing results. I felt like a new person, and every day that passed, I had something more to hold onto, because I saw more results, and I was feeling better every single day.

Shane: So you were getting on the scales every day to look at the progress?

Leslie: I actually did. I tell people to hide the scales and don't look. But there's something deep inside of you that can't seem to help it.

Shane: Leslie, to be honest with you, I also give that advice, but during my first seven-day reboot, which was January 2010, I weighed myself every morning, and I made notes. I still have that notebook and I can see every day what I wrote. For me, it really helped that I could see that progress and it kind of powered me on to the next day, where I could see that it was working. I said, "Wow, I dropped two pounds. I'll keep up with this. It's working." When I was at Camp Reboot in the summer with Joe, we didn't have access to weighing scales because we were staying in dormitory-style cabins.

So you got weighed on a Sunday night and then you got through to Friday, and it was a great surprise to see everyone and how much weight they lost along with inches from their waists and so forth. But that was fine for me, because it was about my tenth cleanse. But I really think for my first one, to keep myself going, I really needed to see the scales.

Leslie: You know another thing I suggest doing is to take a before picture and an after picture. Go three, four, five days, or whatever you want, and even if you're not finished, take another one. Compare them and you can see a difference. You can really see a difference and keep on going. I've got several pictures that I took throughout my journey and they just inspired me.

Shane: I think that's great advice. I wouldn't have believed it before I did my first juice fast, but just five to seven days can have such a big difference, not just in terms of looks. I also journaled. I wrote every day about the differences I experienced. For the first three days, I'll be honest, I felt like crap. But after that, it was like day four, I remember having all this energy, and I wrote about it, and that also helped me. It wasn't just that physical change that I was starting to notice or numbers on the scales. It was also "How do I feel today?" And I remember my sleep after day three was just amazing.

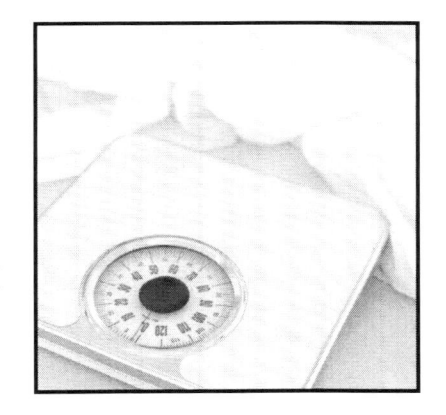

Leslie: The first three days of a fast, you're not going to feel good, so people need to be prepared for that. It's not all fun and games in the beginning. You're going to feel bad.

Shane: I'm really glad to hear you say that, Leslie, because I know a lot of people fail on day one, two, or three, because they don't understand detox, especially for people who are trying this for the first time, if their diets have been very bad and not very clean eating. I started my juice fast probably with the worst hangover ever, because it was New Year's Day, and clearly your body is going to react to that. It's the same way that if you've been drinking five or six cups of coffee a day, your body is going to say, "Whoa, where is my caffeine?" and that's going to have a really painful effect on your body.

But what Leslie and I will tell you is that once you get to day three, four, or five, the abundance of energy and the mental clarity is so worth going through those dark first couple of days. And I love the fact that in Joe's movie, he didn't sugarcoat that. You saw him on his bed in the hotel, absolutely raving in agony, hating it, and that's not cool to look at. And we all have to put ourselves through that in order to get to the other side. So for those of you who might have caffeine or detox withdrawals, or you're feeling like crap, please stick with it, because the benefits are worth it. And when you get to day four or five, you'll be laughing about it. Right, Leslie?

Leslie: That is true. That is very, very true.

Shane: During your first detox, did you have an "aha" moment? When did things first click for you? You thought, "This is working! This is really cool!"

Leslie: Things started to click for me as my fast progressed, and I watched every single food documentary I could get my hands on. Because you get to a point, maybe after you're over that sick spell at first, where you're twittering your fingers, and kind of get bored in a way. So I think watching documentaries gives you something to focus on and more inspiration, because they teach you so much.

I eventually also started to research everything I could on the subject and gained a lot of knowledge to carry on with after I finished my fast. I also created a plan for what steps I wanted to take to change my life.

Shane: I think that is superb advice, Leslie. Are there any documentaries that you recommend?

Leslie: One of my favorites is *Food, Inc.* I think that is a really well-made movie, and it's really interesting. On the lighter side, in a way, I like *May I Be Frank.* I will say it's got some bad language in it. But the movie shows an amazing journey.

Shane: If Leslie is recommending it, it will be well worth watching.

Leslie: Yeah, it's a great story.

Shane: One of the reasons that I really support your idea is it's not just about the green juice you're putting in your body. Angie and I often talk about the mental juice, which I actually think is more important, because you need to also put positive thoughts into your mind. For instance, you might want to watch *Food, Inc.,* or *Forks over Knives,* or other films so you're putting really good ideas into your mind. When you watch them, they really increase your chances of being successful in your detox.

Another thing I found was that if you watch television shows, you won't even notice what's happening on the show. You'll see the burger that's on the dinner table. I'm a huge fan of James Bond, and I remember watching a few of those movies to try to take my mind off the fast. And there is Roger Moore having a sumptuous feast in an Indian palace, so I had to stop. Now when I do cleanses, I watch documentaries because it's so important.

Leslie: I don't watch commercials, especially in the evenings. Evenings are one of the hardest times, for me anyway. You sit down to watch TV, and you've got one food commercial after another. It's just ridiculous. Your mouth starts watering, so turn the TV off.

Shane: My other tip is to go buy the physical copy of *Fat, Sick and Nearly Dead.* Joe Cross shot something like 500 hours for that movie, which is only one-and-a-half hours long. So he's got a lot of extra content that didn't make the film. You can see other people who did a Reboot that didn't make the final cut. There is a wonderful scene in a Laundromat with a little boy and his very obese mother and a discussion that Joe has while she's doing his laundry. So that's a recommendation to buy the physical copy, because online you can't get access to the bonus content.

Leslie: That's true. I actually bought the DVD so that I could watch that, and I ended up giving it to my doctor before I got to watch the extra footage. So I actually have missed out of that.

Shane: Oh, you need to go get it. At the summer Camp Reboot, they were going to do a showing of the movie again, but Joe said, "Let's look at the bonus content. A lot of people haven't seen that, and there are some really powerful scenes in the bonus content." So that's a little tip to buy the DVD.

Leslie, you have a wonderful family. Was that a challenge for you—going on a juice fast while people around you were eating?

Leslie: Not really. Once I reached a certain point, failure wasn't an option for me. I took myself away from the mainstream of food in the house when the kids were eating for the first three or four days. Once I got past that, it was more therapeutic for me to cook, which I enjoyed. I did so much more cooking when I fasted than on a normal day.

Shane: And why do you say failure wasn't an option? Can you explain to us what you mean by that?

Leslie: Once I set my mind to something, I'm going to do it. I'm just hardheaded, and I'm going to do it. I don't allow myself to find excuses or talk myself out of something. I'm not going to fail at it. I get my mind set, and that's what I'm going to do.

Shane: So what was the biggest challenge for you personally, particularly in the early days of your first juice fast?

Leslie: I think the biggest challenge was probably me. I had to fight myself as I almost tried to talk myself out of fasting. I heard that voice inside me that says to eat the last piece of pizza in the refrigerator, or it's going to spoil. Or I'll look in the cabinet and it's the initial mental part of telling myself or rationalizing why I can cheat. I think I was the biggest challenge during my first fast, of course.

Shane: That really resonates with me, because I have to empty all of my cupboards. Even though I've done 10 or 11 of these cleanses now, I have to empty any treats or other items out of my cupboards, because you do have that devil on your shoulder that says, "Oh, you can have those peanuts. That doesn't count." Or like you were saying with the pizza, no one is going to know. It's only one bit of pizza. So I have to empty the kitchen of anything like that, although, like you were saying, I'm fighting myself.

Leslie: I always have to make sure that if there's anything that I really love, it's got to go. I can't even start.

Shane: I agree with that approach. Did you have any specific cravings during your first detox? Was there anything that you were really wanting?

Leslie: Well, more out of habit, I really crave a good cold beer. I mean it's just kind of a habit, and I'm honest about that. And I love peanut butter and jelly on white bread—I should eat it on wheat. After a few days, the cravings subside, just like when you stop smoking. Certain things still trigger that desire, but you just have to kind of set it aside, and it will pass.

Shane: I think that's really good advice. It is the mental strategy, the mental defense that you have to set up to say, no. It's only five days. What I found was the more that I got into the fast, the less I craved unhealthy stuff and instead I craved greens. I remember really craving steamed Brussels sprouts with chili pepper. I never craved that in my life! But on day five or six, I'm saying to myself, "As soon as I can eat again, I'm having steamed Brussels sprouts." People don't believe you. But everyone I speak to tells me the same thing. Your cravings change to healthier foods.

Leslie: Definitely. I didn't want to put anything in my body that could mess up the 30 days that I had invested. You don't want to do that, so you try to keep it clean. And I think that you should not deprive yourself of certain things when you're done, because when you deprive, you restrict things. Instead, you just choose foods in moderation. But you can tell yourself, if I get through this, I can have this occasionally.

Shane: Never say never. Wow, that's so important, and I know a lot of people who are hesitant because they don't want to give up A, B, and C. It's not about giving those things up, but your body might feel really good if you do. My skin is great. My hair is great. I have much more energy. I don't want to put all of that crap back in. However, I allow myself a splurge meal once a week. I will go and have Mexican food on a Friday night, because there is no point in restricting yourself.

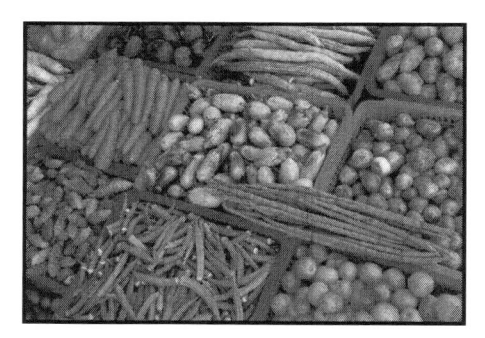

Did you receive any negative feedback from friends, family, coworkers, or anything when you were going through your first fast?

Leslie: Well, I try not to let any negativity into my life. I keep myself full of positivity, that way, there won't be any room to let negative thoughts come in. When it comes to juicing, there is not much debate, because the way I see it, I'm right. I've done the research. I've done the science on it, and there is no negative to it. This works.

Shane: It does work. And for those of you who are going through this the first time, you will probably have conflict from friends and family. You'll have conflict from within yourself. So take the words of successful juicers who are sharing that juicing works.

Leslie, what advice, based on your experience, would you give to someone starting their detox? Imagine someone who's never done this before. They're on day one, what advice would you give them?

Leslie: I would tell them, "Do not let it overwhelm you."

Shane: How do you mean?

Leslie: A lot of people think that you have to have all these recipes and you have to do everything point-to-point-to point. And you have to have all of these rules and guidelines, but there's a lot of information out there. Take time to do your research before you start. Watch the movie *Fat, Sick and Nearly Dead.* Those are the best tools I think to keep it simple. Have fun with it, and make it realistic to your life so that it can be a permanent change.

Shane: I actually love your idea of freestyling, because that's what keeps it interesting. If you're only allowed to have a chickpea salad for all meals for five days a week, you're going to get terribly bored. Whereas if you can mix things up, you can keep it interesting and varied. For instance, on Tuesday night, I'm going to make a juice with a sweet potato. The beautiful thing with juicing is there are very few rules.

I mean there is advice such as "Don't juice with an orange with a peel on" for instance, but there are very few rules to follow. And it really is fun to experiment. You might make a juice that is revolting, and on the other hand, you might make a juice that you like. For me, carrot, apple, ginger is still my all-time favorite juice. Out of all of the wonderful juices that I've had, that's the one that gets me every time.

Leslie: We all have our little favorite ones.

Shane: What's yours? I know you make so many, but is there one that you like?

Leslie: I'm doing the "25 Days of Christmas," and I'm counting down. I've done a different juice for every single day. I kind of like the carrots, apples, and ginger. You can't beat that.

Shane: So what habits did you create during your first detox to really help you succeed? You mentioned that you really strengthened your mind to succeed. Are there any others? For instance, during the juice prep, was there anything around that you did to make sure that you were successful and didn't fall off the wagon?

Leslie: What I did was to make sure in the afternoon to sip hot herbal tea. You get the satisfaction of having the warmth in your body rather than the cold juice, but it doesn't hurt your fast. And I had gum to help pacify the need to chew, and it helps with the way your mouth feels. You know about ten minutes after you drink a Mean Green, that's what I call the fuzzy tongue syndrome, because it feels like you've got that coat in your mouth.

Shane: Those are some great tips! Leslie, in terms of people wanting to follow you online, you have a very active Facebook group, which is Juicing for Dummies, right?

Leslie: Yes, it sure is.

Shane: I highly recommend, especially for those of you on your first cleanse, to take a look at the Juicing for Dummies Facebook Group page. There is a ton of information on there. Leslie works really hard to give free information. There are also a lot of people on there who have been very successful, and also a lot of first timers. You're also on Twitter, right Leslie?

Leslie: Yes, I am, juicing4dummies.

Shane: Leslie, I know your words are going to be helpful, particularly for all of the first-time juicers. Angie and I are really grateful for the work that you do in outreach in terms of juicing and promoting this as a healthy lifestyle.

Leslie: Thank you. I want to wish everybody reading this good luck! Stick with it, and like I said, have fun. You're going to see the results, and you're going to feel great.

Connect with Leslie

Twitter

juicing4dummies

Facebook

https://www.facebook.com/JuicingForDummies

Get your free copy of *How to Get Started with Juicing* and receive free email juice coaching (but not spam—that's not healthy).

Sign up at www.juicinghabits.com.

JUICING RADIO

Shane and Angie invite you to listen to a juicing success story every week on Juicing Radio.

Sign up for updates and never miss an episode at JuicingRadio.com.

Always Motivational and Informative!

by lsulli5

Love this podcast. I always learn something new and leave feeling motivated. I enjoy the fact that the interviews are with people who have been through the journey and have been successful both mentally and physically. Shane, you are a great interviewer, thanks! And Angie, you are inspiration and I love the recipes.

Chapter 4
Angie
Shares Visions of Success

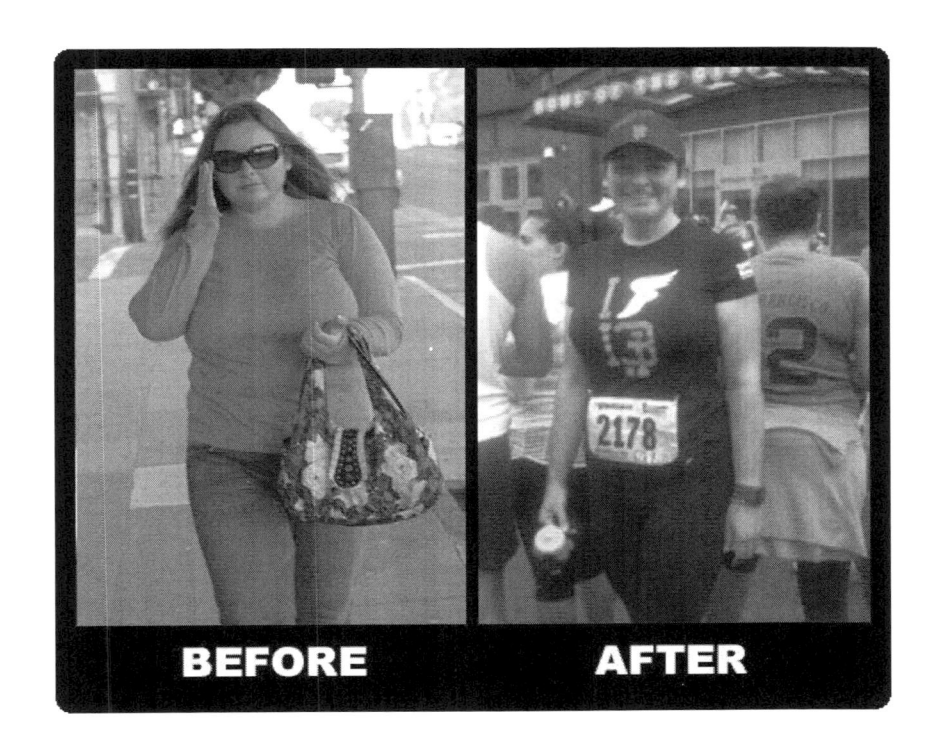

BEFORE **AFTER**

Shane: It is my pleasure to introduce to you a familiar voice to those of you who are regular listeners to Juicing Radio. Hello, Angie.

Angie: Hi, Shane!

Shane: Angie lost 86 pounds through juicing. She completed two half marathons and when she started out on this whole journey, she couldn't run for one minute nonstop. She's appeared in a commercial, advertising *Fat, Sick and Nearly Dead,* which was shown in the United States for the first time on December 29, 2013.

I think the amazing thing about Angie's story is that she was doing really well—she was running, she was juicing, she was losing weight—and then, unfortunately, Angie broke her ankle. She was on crutches and unable to work out for more than a year. Most of us probably would have reverted to snacks, chocolate, ice cream and put the weight back on. But Angie continued to lose weight, which is amazing.

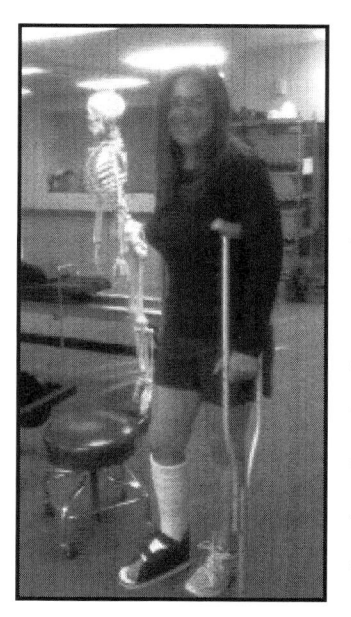

Angie: Thank you so much!

Shane: Let's talk about your first juice fast. What made you start a ten-day juice fast?

Angie: I was on vacation in Hawaii, and when I got back I realized that for most of my vacation I was consumed with negative thoughts about how uncomfortable I was on the beach in a bathing suit. I was just really preoccupied, and I realized that I wasn't enjoying my life. I mean here I was in one of the most beautiful places on Earth and it was so peaceful, but I couldn't really focus on enjoying it because I was preoccupied. So I decided I needed to do something, and I decided to do a ten-day juice fast. I ended the fast on my birthday, and I never looked back. It was probably the most loving gift I've ever given to myself

Shane: How do you mean?

Angie: There's a domino effect that happened after I finished my ten-day juice fast. I lost about seventeen pounds in ten days. Juice is almost like a magical elixir. When you start to feel better and lighter, and things start to shift a little bit, it affects other areas of your life. So when I started the ten-day juice fast, I wasn't exercising, I had high blood pressure, and I wasn't sleeping well. It's amazing what you can do when you start getting a good night's sleep, and your body starts to become healthier. You feel better, and when you feel better you do better. My relationships improved, my mood improved, I started exercising, and I ended up getting two promotions at work. It really impacted all areas of my life, and it all started with juicing.

Shane: Wow. That's something that we are learning a great deal about with all the different juicing success stories. It's not just about the weight loss, but there are lots of other benefits to going through juice fasts. So when you started the ten-day juice fast, what program did you follow?

Angie: I didn't have a specific program that I followed. I kind of put it together myself. I read your Juicing Starter Guide, and I read some recipes from Running on Juice, and I found some ideas in recipe books and online. But I had been juicing, one juice a day for a little while, so I'd experimented quite a bit. I knew which juices worked for me and the ones that I really enjoyed. So I focused on those and I created my own program, and that was what worked for me.

Shane: That's fascinating, Angie. All of the people we've interviewed for this series actually did what we call freestyle juicing. Basically they had Joe Cross's Mean Green juice, and they had their own green juices they were making. It seems that everyone actually just said, "Okay, I'm going to be experimenting and come up with my own regimen." And I think a part of that is because when a lot of our success story participants were starting their juicing program, Joe's site wasn't that functional. He didn't have his programs on there yet, and there weren't that many juicing programs anyway. But I think there's something more to it. Why do you think the success stories in this book started freestyle juicing?

Angie: Well, I think everyone is different, and one program won't work for everybody. People are entering into it at different states. I know that when I first started juicing, I couldn't tolerate beets. Everyone has different tastes, so you can kind of gravitate toward recipes that you really enjoy and that work for you as an individual. Like I said, one-size-fits-all programs don't necessarily work for everyone.

Shane: That's why I do like what Joe Cross is doing with the Guided Reboot, where you have coaches able to assist you. Back in the day, it was like "Have this juice four times a day and you're done with it." Now you can talk to someone and say, for instance, "Look, I can't tolerate celery, or beets, or kale." There's actually someone who you can talk to and get some good nutritional advice from. Also there are lots of communities out there to help you. There's RunningOnJuice.com. There's JuicingRadio.com. There are Facebook groups, such as Juicing for Dummies, so there are lots of groups where you can go and talk with people. In the past they weren't in existence for some of us. I know when I started juicing Joe's movie wasn't even out. I had one book by Jason Vale (known as the Juice Master) and that was it.

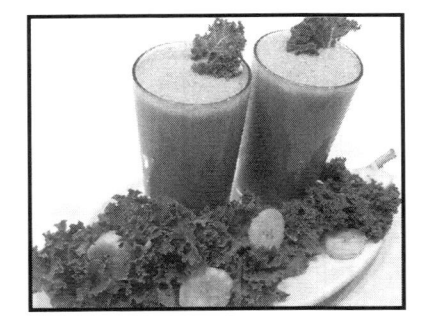

Angie: It's really a whole new world! There's so much online support and so much educational material with lots of great tips. People starting to juice now actually have a huge advantage.

Shane: But I still like what you're saying, which is basically to come up with your own juice recipes that work for you. Brian, one of our other success stories, said that he tried to make his juice to the formula of 80 percent veggies and 20 percent fruit. I think as long as you try to stick with that formula, you'll do well. I made a juice of pineapple, grapes, and ginger, and I thought, "That sounds a bit different, I'll give it a go." It turned out to have about 600 calories. I know we shouldn't get hung up on the calories, but that was lot more calories in a juice than I thought it would be.

Angie: Yeah.

Shane: But it was all fruit, so that's why

Angie: I think you bring up an interesting point about sweet juices—juices that are kind of sugar heavy. I think people get caught up in doing it the "right" way—and yes, the goal should be an 80/20 ratio or 60/40 ratio—but some people aren't quite there yet. I know when I started, I wasn't. I couldn't do veggie juices that were that veggie heavy and sometimes I would add a little extra apple, or a little extra pear, or coconut water to sweeten it up a bit so I could tolerate it. That's where I was at the time. Eventually, I was able to move forward and get into more veggie-heavy juices, but you have to be willing to accept where you are when you start and create your own program for that. So I think that modifying the juice to suit your own taste so you actually drink it is really important.

Shane: Great advice, Angie. Especially if it's your first juice fast, maybe you're closing your eyes and knocking the stuff back, but you've gotta make it work for you. That's the real important thing, and you can always work to get that percentage right. This is the thing, and you might find this hard to believe right now, but the more you juice, the more your taste buds will change and you'll reach that 80/20. Sometimes I will have 100 percent green juice, which, in fact, I've only started enjoying in the last year. Before that I couldn't really tolerate it.

So, Angie, were you scared during your first juice fast?

Angie: I wasn't really scared. I guess concerned would be a more accurate word. I was a little concerned about my energy levels and being able to function at my job, and just function in life.

Shane: What was your job at the time?

Angie: I worked for a nonprofit agency that provides mental health services for very vulnerable children and their families.

Shane: So it's a really stressful job.

Angie: Yes, a very stressful job. It's a job where people's lives are in your hands, and it's very important to be 100 percent all the time. So that was one of my concerns as I tried to set myself up for success, because I knew that the detox symptoms would happen more in the beginning.

I started the juice fast on a weekend when I knew I could rest. I didn't schedule anything and I had a little bit of time to get through those detox symptoms. By Day 4, I'm actually really thrilled because that's when the energy surge comes for me on the fast. The detox symptoms start to wane and you start to feel human—even a little superhuman—at that point. It's different for everyone, but Day 4 is my favorite.

I guess going back to your question, my major concern was my energy level and being able to function at my job.

Shane: I think a lot of people of people can relate, and that's a really smart tip to start on a weekend. But for those of you who need to start on a different day, don't worry about it. Get on with it. Don't give up—keep on going through.

Angie: If you're already on Day 4, you're in the clear.

Shane: Angie makes a really good point. You're going to struggle the first few days. This is what I love about Joe's movie—the first couple of days he's in a bad way, he's kind of hiding under his bedclothes in his hotel.

I rebooted over Christmas week and the first one or two days, I was like a bear with a sore head. But I've done fourteen reboots in the past few years, and I've learned that it's just part of the journey. But once you push through to Day 3, and like Angie said Day 4, your energy levels are through the roof. Why do you think your first detox was so successful?

Angie: I think a big part of the success of my first detox was that I'd been juicing one juice a day for a while, for several months, so I was familiar with the machine. I was familiar with what I liked and what I didn't like, and I think that had a big part of my success. Preparation is also part of it and the other part was my mindset. I decided that by any means necessary this was going to happen for me. And it was a decision like no other I'd ever made before. It was backed up by some radical action, and failure was not an option. So I think my mental state at the time was optimistic. I reached out to people who I knew were healthy, who'd been juicing before. I reached out to people who were into exercise. I read positive things. I listened to positive things. I watched *Fat, Sick and Nearly Dead.* I really filled myself with positivity and visions of success.

Shane: So it's interesting that you just mentioned that failure wasn't an option. Leslie, another of our successful juicers, said the same thing on Day 1. So that is common with people who have been successful with juicing. You have to commit mentally that failure is not an option, and you're going to push through this. Because you know there are low moments when you want to give up. But, if you say to yourself, "Look, failure is not an option! I'm going to do X days!" Then you have to resolve to do that.

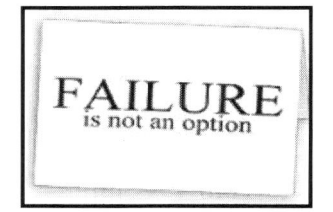

Angie, during your first juice fast, did you have an "aha" moment? Was there any time when you said, "This is clicking for me, this is good, I'm on the right track."

Angie: Probably on Day 4, or soon after Day 4, when my energy started to really increase. I had a hard time right before I started my juice fast looking in the mirror. And I was a little bit in denial about what I had become and how I'd gotten there. There was a part that was a little scary but it was also empowering when I took responsibility for where I was and that I had gotten myself there. But the part that was really empowering was that if I got myself there, I can get myself out. And each day that went by I just felt stronger, and the more I did something that was good for me and the better I felt, the more I thought was possible for me. So I think my "aha" moment was taking responsibility for my condition, and then feeling empowered to be able to do something about it and change it.

Shane: Wow, that's good stuff, Angie. During your first detox, did you have any specific cravings?

Angie: Yes. I do love a good cup of espresso in the morning, and I've had that habit for a long time. First thing when I would wake up, I would have an espresso, so that was definitely an adjustment. I would often replace that with a wheatgrass juice, which is kind of Mother Nature's espresso, and a much healthier alternative.

Shane: Wow. Anything else? Because you're a fan of ice cream too, right?

Angie: I do love ice cream and I love salt-and-pepper potato chips. I didn't have a ton of cravings for those things, but I go there when I want to celebrate, or for emotional eating. Those are definitely a treat!

Shane: When you were going through your juice fasts, either your first one or consecutive ones, did you receive any negative feedback from friends and family?

Angie: I did receive some negative feedback. When I would take my green juice to work, there were a few people who would stop me or say, "What's that? What are you drinking?" And I remember one coworker stopped me and said, "Do you know that's green?" And what's really funny is that I adore this particular person, and I got a message from him that he just bought his first juicer. So he wrote to ask me for juice recipes.

Shane: Wow.

Angie: So, that's full circle! Even though there are naysayers, he watched my whole transformation from the very beginning, and couldn't understand why I would drink something that was green. But he saw it all and now he's actually going to start juicing.

Shane: This brings up something else. We are all very positive commercials for juicing. Something happened on *Good Morning America* where some people were criticizing juicing—talking about the high amounts of sugar, the high calories, and everything else. People wrote to me about this and my reply was that the shows never ask people like you and me, who have juiced off a lot of weight, to actually counter these arguments.

So I hope that the next time the topic is juicing, someone will contact us and invite one of our seven success stories onto the show, and we can counter the so-called experts, who think that this is a fad and that it is dangerous. I'm getting quite passionate about this now, because I'm angry when I read or see negative remarks about juicing. And I get that negativity sells. But the shows don't get people on to counter that and say,

"Well, hang on, you lost 86 pounds, you've got promoted twice, you've run half marathons, you said it yourself, it's the most loving gift you could give yourself." Instead you've got these so-called experts "warning" people by saying, "Oh, the sugar's too high in a juice."

Angie: You know what, it's really infuriating. The sugar's high in juice compared to what? Compared to a venti frappuccino? No. You're doing something that's densely nutritious and if you need to start off with it being a little on the sweet side, at least you're getting it into your body. The alternatives are not great.

Shane: Absolutely. For any of the media organizations that might be interested, please contact us and we'll gladly provide you with names and phone numbers of people who will come on your show and talk about the positive effects of juicing. Anyway, that was completely unscripted and not planned, so let's get back to you, Angie.

What advice would you give to someone who is ready or just starting their detox?

Angie: Well, I'd give a few words of advice. One is to really do a lot of preparation, but don't get too concerned about being perfect. Do your best with what you have available. If you only have the funds to do one juice a day, then do one juice a day. If you can only borrow a juicer, do that. Just start. Just start the journey.

Shane: Angie, that's music to my ears. I thought you were going to quote my favorite Morrissey song, "Do your best and don't worry."

Angie: Do your best and don't worry. I've heard that song quite a bit because of you, and now I've grown to love it, because people can get caught up in perfection paralysis. So you really just need to move forward and not worry too much about the details.

Shane: In what? What was that technical label?

Angie: Perfection paralysis is when you're so worried about doing it absolutely right, that you end up doing nothing at all.

Shane: That's a new one for me.

Angie: So, don't get wrapped up in doing it exactly perfect. Just start. And you know what? It will be perfect. When you start, things will unfold. Before I did the ten-day juice fast, I started with one juice a day, found recipes that I liked and it led to the next step and to the next step. It's really an evolution, and everybody goes at their own pace, so don't worry about doing it exactly the way I've done it, or exactly the way Joe's done it, or Shane's done it. You have to find your own path and use other people's wisdom to guide you, but you also have internal wisdom. You know yourself better than anyone else. And if you start to think about it, you'll know what will work for you. So start to analyze your behavior a little bit, and think about where you might have messed up in the past, and don't beat yourself up about it, but learn from that, and change your course a little bit. There's a quote that I really love by Marianne Williamson. She says, "Our deepest fear is not that we are inadequate, our deepest fear is that we are powerful beyond measure."

Shane: Wow, that's pretty profound.

Angie: I think it's so profound, and when you're able listen to your inner wisdom and what you know will work for you, you're going to be successful. It's just kind of tapping into that and trusting it. That theme really goes into taking responsibility for yourself. If you believe that you're inadequate and that you can't do it, well that kind of takes the pressure off, right? There's nothing I can do about it. But if you are powerful beyond measure, you can change it.

Shane: What habits did you create to really help you succeed on your first juice fast?

Angie: One of the habits that I did on my first juice fast was to make quite a bit of juice in the morning. So I would start off with at least three juices in the morning, so they were all ready to go. So when I got a little hungry or ready for another juice, I didn't actually have to make it at the time, it was ready. That really helped.

One of the other habits I got into was taking a little walk, even if I didn't feel like it. It's important to move your body just a little bit, even if you can just go around the block, just move your body.

Making sure I went to bed early was another thing that was really helpful.

I also planned to do something. When you're not planning meals, eating, or cooking, it frees up a lot of time. So I would do other things for myself that were self soothing or self care. I took a lavender bath every day. So plan to do something nice for yourself that doesn't have to do with eating.

Shane: So there are some really good habits from Angie. We hope you continue to inspire people when it comes to juicing and changing their lives for good. And we really hope to see you out there in your running shoes again soon, because I know how much you enjoyed running and how much it helped you burn stress and appreciate life. And maybe I'll get to see you in New York at some stage, and you can kick my backside running around Central Park.

Angie: Oh, that's been a dream of mine for a long time. Not only running in Central Park, but kicking your backside!

Angie lost 86 pounds

and kept it off despite not being able to exercise. She answers the question "What do juicers eat?" and shares her recipes on WhatJuicersEat.com.

Sign up and never miss a recipe again!

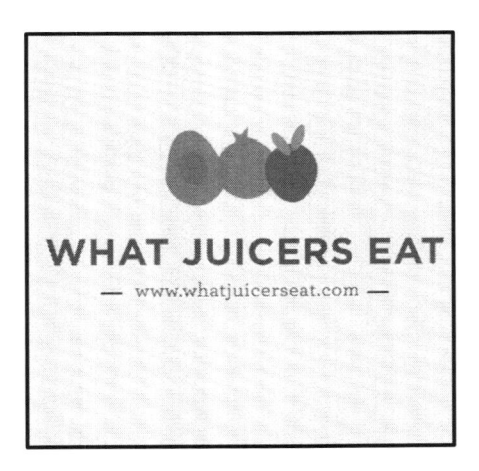

Get your free copy of
How to Get Started with Juicing
**and receive free email juice coaching
(but not spam—that's not healthy).**

Sign up at www.juicinghabits.com

JUICING RADIO

Shane and Angie invite you to listen to a juicing success story every week on Juicing Radio.

Sign up for updates and never miss an episode at JuicingRadio.com.

Great Show from a Living Testimonial

by Sam of TipsOfTheScale.com

Juicing Radio is a fantastic resource for anyone curious about juicing. Shane and crew are extremely knowledgeable, they walk the walk, and their passion for the topic shines through.

Chapter 5

Brian

Determined to Make a Change

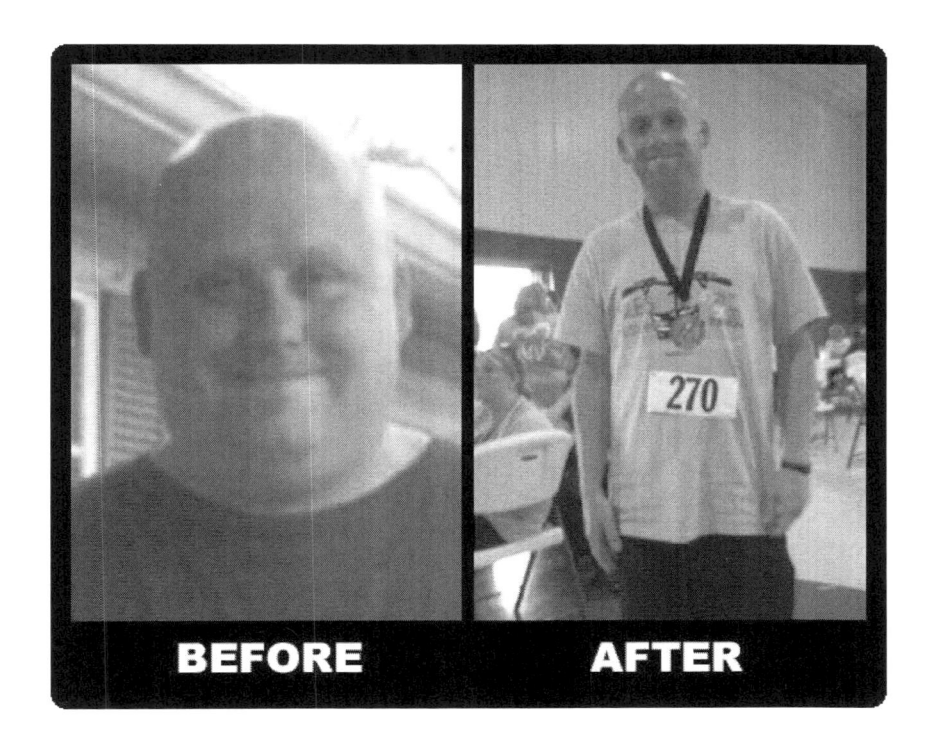

BEFORE **AFTER**

Shane: Hi, Brian. If I've got my data correct, you juice fasted for about 10 months and lost 165 pounds, right?

Brian: That's correct, Shane.

Shane: Fantastic. So can you explain to us what made you start your very first juice fast?

Brian: I was just really overweight and my health was really poor, and I knew I needed to make a change. I saw Joe's film (Fat, Sick and Nearly Dead) and I thought, "Well, this is the way to try."

Shane: How overweight were you? Do you mind sharing what your weight was when you started?

Brian: I weighed 350 pounds.

Shane: Wow, so you actually lost half your body weight?

Brian: Exactly half my body weight.

Shane: That's incredible. And what juicing program did you follow when you first started?

Brian: When I first started, there wasn't a program. I just copied what I saw in the film.

Shane: So you freestyle juiced? You didn't follow a written program or program out of a book. You just kind of thought, "Okay, well, Joe's drinking that Mean Green, so I'm going to drink that mainly?

Brian: Yeah, I stuck with mostly green juices. I didn't follow his Mean Green exactly, as every once in a while I would throw something different in. I just tried to keep it mostly 80 percent vegetable and 20 percent fruit.

Shane: That's a fantastic suggestion, and it's certainly one we always share with people new to juicing. At the start it can sometimes be difficult to do the 80/20 mix. So if you have to start at 50/50, start at that, then gradually work down to 60/40, 70/30, and then the sweet spot of 80/20. Now, when you started your juice fast, you didn't have a juicer, right?

Brian: No, I just had a blender, and my first juices were pretty awful.

Shane: Do you remember one in particular that was bad?

Brian: The first one was really bad just because I didn't blend it enough—I just hit pulse. I didn't know what I was doing and just gave it a few seconds. Then I put it in a jug and waited until the next morning. I think the first one I had was Granny Smith apple, some kind of pear, celery, kale, and probably cabbage—just a lot of green fruits and vegetables. And the next morning, I poured it into a glass, and it just kind of plopped out and looked like bad milk.

Shane: Yeah.

Brian: I brought my children into the kitchen to watch me drink my first juice and had to fight it down, gagging, but I knew I had to do it. So I was able just to power that one and keep going and just kind of learn along the way.

Shane: I think what's great with your story, Brian, is that you continued. For anyone who wants to start juicing now, we're very blessed to have the Reboot with Joe Cross program, which has free plans on the website. There are also YouTube videos, websites, podcasts, and a lot of resources [See Bibliography and Resources at the end of this book] to actually be successful on your first juice fast.

I've got to be honest with you, Brian. If I had made that juice in a blender, waited a day, and then drank it, maybe I wouldn't have carried on. So I think it's really incredible that you did.

Brian: Thank you, Shane.

Shane: So think back to the first week of your juice fast. You've decided, "I'm going to juice. I've watched the movie. I'm going to change my life for good." Were you scared?

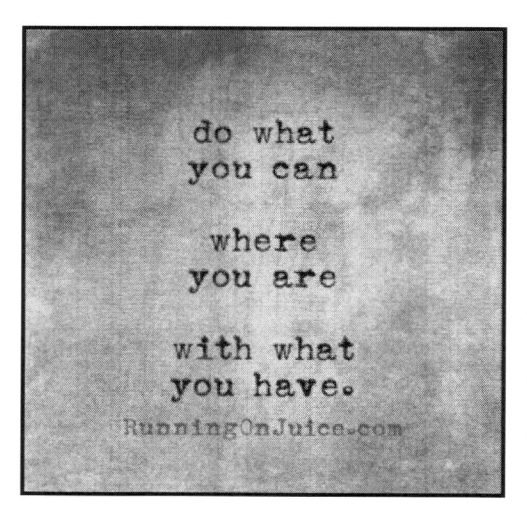

> do what you can
>
> where you are
>
> with what you have.
>
> RunningOnJuice.com

Brian: Not at all. I think if I was afraid of anything, it was that maybe what I saw in the film was some kind of a scam and wouldn't work. I had failed miserably before, so there was a little bit of a fear of failure. But after the first week, I was down 15 pounds, my energy was through the roof, and all the fear was gone. I mean, it was like just kind of rolling downhill.

Shane: For those of you who might be on your first juice fast, this is something that all our juicing experts want to really stress—the first few days are horrible, particularly if your diet has been bad, and then you suddenly make the jump into juicing. But like Brian is saying, by the end of his first week his energy was through the roof, and he'd lost 15 pounds. It really is worth trudging through those first few horrible days, right, Brian?

Brian: Exactly. And you just give it four days, at least four days, because the first three days you can feel like crap. But you want to at least give it a fair try so that you can get to that point where you can feel that rush of energy.

Shane: And did you know anybody else, apart from Joe in the movie, who had juiced before?

Brian: I had a friend who told me about the movie, and she had juiced, but I don't think it was for any length of time. Out of all the people that I know, I was the first person who had actually gone on a juice fast.

Shane: I can relate to that. When I tried my first juice fast in 2008, I got talked out of it because I didn't know anybody else who'd done it. It was before the movie and there wasn't much support. So please listen to all the experts in this book, because we were where you are now. I didn't know anybody who juiced. Now you have trust in the movie, and you should have trust in the experts.

So, Brian, during that first week, what do you think was the biggest challenge for you?

Brian: The biggest challenge for me was cooking for my children in the evenings. My children were in school at that time, so I could go all day long and I was fine, but in the evening when I had to cook supper for them, and I was just trying to stay strong and drink the juice, that was the biggest challenge for me.

Shane: How did you overcome that?

Brian: I had a juice ready so that if I felt the need for something, I could get the juice. At that time I was drinking the same juice, just some kind of a green juice. Now I tell people to have a juice that you really like for that time of day, even if it's more fruit or something that you can just reach for that can be a treat, because then you think in a different way. There could be more apple in that juice or some kind of berry that you really like. Just have it ready for your weakest point of the day. So I would make food for my children. I would plate it and give it to them, and then go into another room or go on the porch, go outside and walk a little bit while they ate, and just remove the temptation.

Shane: That's really good advice. During that week, did you have any specific cravings?

Brian: I don't think so. I know the second week, I was watching the film with my brother and my mother, and my brother decided that the thing to do while he was watching the film would be eat pizza. So that was a torturous two hours, because anything with melted cheese was my temptation. So that was kind of hard. But going through it, you can feel proud, and I didn't give in.

Shane: Sure. There is a lot of pride in that. I mean, to be there when someone's eating pizza in front of you. It's like the lady in the movie—she sat there with her green juice and her husband is eating steak and ribs. I always think that's a lot of determination not to fall off the wagon.

Brian: When I was early in the program, I liked to seek out those moments.

Shane: You did?

Brian: Because I knew if I could make it through that, then I had it conquered.

Shane: Interesting. So you used that as strength through adversity?

Brian: Exactly.

Shane: When you were going through the early part of the juicing, did you receive any negative feedback from friends and family?

Brian: A little bit from my family, but it wasn't too much. It was just from a point of concern. "Are you going to get enough?" or "Is this healthy?" Before I started juicing, my skin tone looked almost like a zombie. I had a real grey complexion. But then my skin tone changed so fast. I looked healthy. I looked alive. My physician knew about juicing. He had seen the movie and told me, "This is great. This is one of the best things you can do for yourself." So I was able to relay that message to my family.

Shane: You're so lucky to have a doctor who's that progressive, knew about juicing, and was able to give you that mental reinforcement that you were doing a good thing, Brian.

Brian: I felt really lucky.

Shane: So if you were speaking to someone who's starting their first juice fast, juice detox, reboot; call it what you will; what advice would you give to that first timer, who's a little nervous, a little scared, not sure if they're going to be able to do it? What would you say to that person?

Brian: I would say, knowing what I know now, "Plan on making a variety of power juices throughout the day, just because you might not be able to tolerate a green juice or everything that's in your green juice. If you can do one that's orange or a red juice, or just try a lot of different things. And try to give it at least four days."

Shane: That's good advice. When you talk about drinking the color of the rainbow, I made a juice the other day, which was from the Reboot site, and I hadn't juiced a sweet potato in ages, and it had two pears and blueberries. You juice the lot and then you stir in some cinnamon, and that was delicious. That was almost like a dessert—a spicy Christmas pie.

Brian: That's one of my favorite juices that you're talking about.

Shane: I would never have thought about juicing a sweet potato.

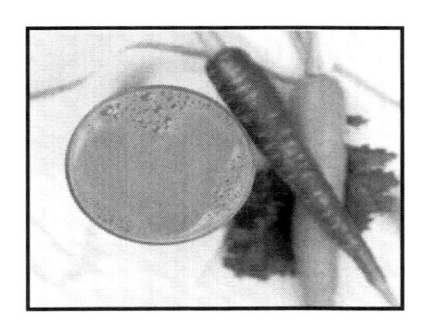

Brian: Oh, it's great. I do it a lot. I like doing a red apple, sweet potato, carrots, and pineapple.

Shane: I bet that's delicious. And it goes back to what you were saying earlier about when you feel you're starting to want to give in—make yourself one of these kind of dessert-like juices that is sweet tasting and will help you through the fast.

Brian: Exactly. You just have to. And I really think you have to go into it with the right mental thought that you know you're going to do this.

Shane: I completely agree with you. What habits did you create? If you remember back to the first juice fast, what kind of lifestyle habits did you create to really help you succeed? You've explained that you would make the juice before you started cooking your kids' dinner, which is a fantastic strategy because then if you have that juice in your hand, you're not going to start picking into whatever you're cooking. But did you create other habits?

Brian: Exercise. I started walking, and after I got to a point where I could run, I started running. But you don't have to run. Just do some kind of exercise, even if it's playing with your children or walking your dog. I really think that those kinds of things help you. When you start to feel weaker, you start to feel hungry. Just take your mind off it. I think that's a really good idea.

Shane: How many days into the fast do you remember that you started exercising?

JUICING RADIO

Shane and Angie invite you to listen to a juicing success story every week on Juicing Radio.

Sign up for updates and never miss an episode at JuicingRadio.com.

Keeps Me on Track

by Skipper1994

There is no better combination than working out while listening to a Juicing Radio podcast. Keeps me focused on my goals. I also love to listen to the podcast while juicing. And I listen to Shane and his guests when I'm feeling on the verge of giving up on my quest for better health and weight loss. Every episode leaves me inspired and ready to pick it up again.

Chapter 6
Nancy
Transforms Her Life to a Wholeness Perspective

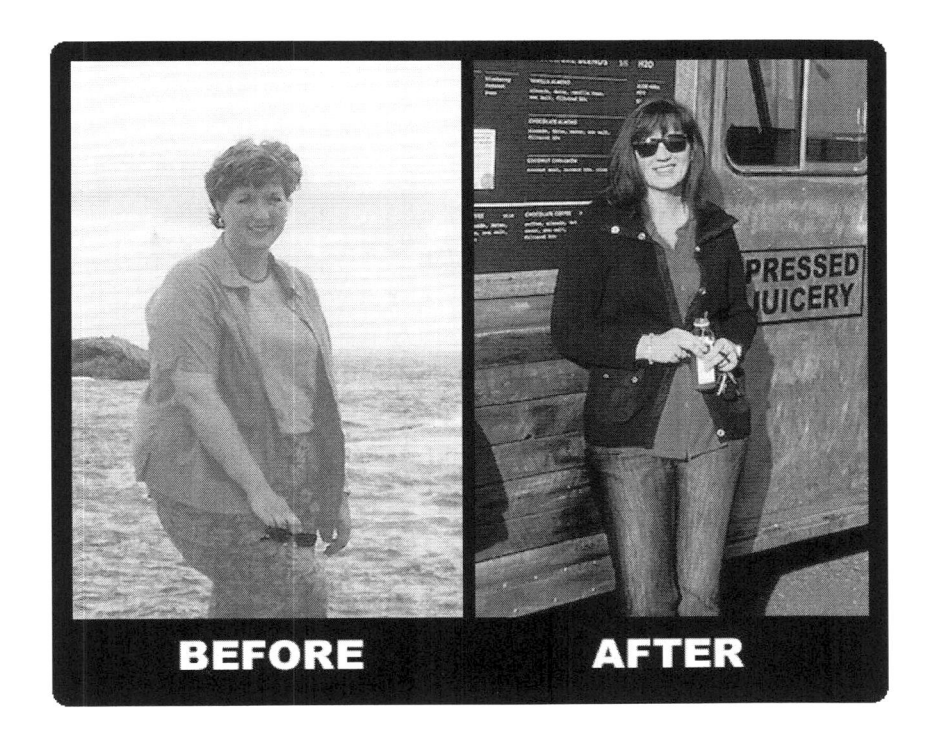

BEFORE AFTER

Shane: Nancy joins us from Los Angeles, California. One of the reasons I wanted to include Nancy in this book is that she's a fairly recent juicer, and within one month, she lost 27 pounds. Overall, she's lost almost 120 pounds through embracing a healthy lifestyle. Welcome, Nancy.

Nancy: Thank you, Shane.

Shane: What was it that made you look to juicing and start a juicing detox? You were doing really well embracing a healthy lifestyle, and then you tried juicing. What made you start?

Nancy: Well, I had a lot of success with eating a mostly plant-based diet, but I sustained a knee injury and it was very painful. I knew that I needed to do something, but it was difficult to exercise. I just felt like if I lost some more weight, it could only help my knee. We're Facebook friends, and I saw that you had posted some things about Juicing Radio. I listened to the podcasts, and I was incredibly inspired by your story, by Angie's story, and others. I felt like I needed to pursue this—that this might be an opportunity for me to reach my final goal on the journey I have been on for the past six years.

I got brave and I decided "I'm going to do this." I contacted you and asked, "Where do I start?" You suggested I watch *Fat, Sick and Nearly Dead,* and it was very inspirational to me. As I was watching, probably the segment that was most impactful was when they were talking about their life expectancy. The one guy says, "I expect to maybe make it to 45," and I'm like, "45, are you crazy?" I want to live to be in my 90s before I say goodbye. I have so much to do in this life. I was shocked that people were saying they'd be done at 45.

Mentally, that just really raised a flag in my mind that I needed to pursue this, as a great option that could help me. The combination of those things was definitely instrumental in making my decision.

Shane: You listened to a couple of success story episodes of Juicing Radio and you watched the Joe Cross movie *Fat, Sick and Nearly Dead,* and you went out and bought yourself a juicer. What program did you follow? What did you then do?

Nancy: The way I operate in my life is when I have decisions to make, things that I want to pursue, whether it's professionally, with my health, or whatever; I really am aggressive about educating myself. You had given me some excellent information. I went to Juicing Radio's website and got some good guidance. I went to Reboot with Joe and got excellent material there. I researched different articles, trying to educate myself, so when I did the detox I could have the best information. Then I could customize and that would be flexible to fit my lifestyle.

Shane: You're starting this juice fast, were you scared when you started it?

Nancy: I wasn't scared, to be honest, but I was very hesitant because I started just a few days before Thanksgiving, and I thought to myself, "You are nuts. You are crazy to start this."

However, I was ready to make that kind of commitment and to really challenge myself to see if I had the discipline to make it through. I wanted to do a fourteen-day fast. At the end of seven days, I could sense my body was "OK, I'm done." I think that's important that juicers are sensitive to what their bodies are telling them. So, I transitioned off my fast. I was very hesitant to start Thanksgiving week, but it ended up being a very empowering experience for me.

Shane: Thanksgiving is a huge deal and a lot of it is centered on food. How did you cope with not eating all that food on Thanksgiving Day?

Nancy: It was really tough, but online I found a picture of a turkey that was arranged and actually made out of fruit. That was my inspiration. I thought, *That's my turkey this year and I'm going to juice.* I did and I was very successful with that detox and the transition off. I was out of town for a few days and when I came back I started my second juice fast. That was just before Christmas, and it was really tough, because I do a lot of holiday baking for people. In the past I've tested the food before I deliver it to people. This year I couldn't, and I was hoping that it tasted good. It was difficult to do that.

Shane: Let's be honest, a juice fast for the first few days is very tough mentally. You get a lot of mental hunger; you get a lot of weird wacky thoughts coming into your mind. Especially on a holiday, when everyone is posting pictures of their meals and I've got my green juice. I was kind of beating myself up about it.

Then I reframed and said, "Shane, this is a really good time to be juicing," because I wasn't with my family and all my friends were out of town, so there was no social commitment. So once I reframed it to actually say, "This is the best week in the year for you, Shane, to do the juice fast because you've got no social distractions," then I felt a lot better.

Nancy: In the past, the food brought a lot of comfort to me and that was part of the problem I dealt with as I gained weight. Then I really realized what I was able to do and it was very rewarding to me. When I made food for others, normally I would have also eaten it. The comfort and happiness I felt I was receiving from that food in the past, actually was replaced when I took the food to people and saw their smiles, their happiness, and the comfort it brought to them.

Part of the biggest success at losing weight was replacing what food brought me as emotional comfort, which was not healthy, and replacing it with other things that brought me happiness and comfort. I really enjoyed seeing the expression on other people's faces when I delivered different treats to them. That's what brought me my comfort and my happiness, my satisfaction, instead of when I used the food as a resource.

Shane: On the back of that, why do you think your first juice fast was successful?

Nancy: You know, I just dove into it, and I just was really committed. It was a combination of determination and realizing it was great, because four days into my first juice fast, I was walking up the stairs in my own condominium. Like I said, I had a really bad knee injury and after the four days, it just registered in my head that my knee wasn't hurting as I was going up the stairs. It was shocking to me. I went in my bedroom, lay on my bed, and started bending my knee. All the stiffness and the pain were just gone. I had been looking at surgery for my knee and I knew that's really a difficult surgery.

I knew the weight loss would help with my knee, but it was amazing to actually have that pain and that stiffness gone. I think it partly the removal of processed grains in my diet and there was less inflammation being generated in my body. I was also getting incredible nutrients from the regular, straight raw juice. I think it was a combination of those things.

Shane: If you read this online or someone on Facebook posted it, you might doubt it. But I know Nancy and she's telling the truth here! I'm very careful on Juicing Radio about discussing the benefits of juicing, because there is so little scientific and empirical evidence. But more and more people are talking about the miraculous effects, if you will, of juicing.

What you're saying is that you walked up the stairs and realized, "Wow, I'm day four on a juice fast and I don't have any knee pain." It's absolutely awesome, so thank you for sharing that with us. What do you think was the biggest challenge, other than being Thanksgiving, for your first juice fast?

Nancy: I usually work from home, so when I started juicing, it was very easy for me to implement and integrate juicing into my lifestyle. But after I transitioned off that first detox, I had to go out of town for some business. Where I went, there were no juice bars and I chose not to take my juicer with me. It was really tough to go without the juices.

Finally, the last day, I found a great juice bar in a nearby city and was thrilled to be able to have some fresh juice. I would say finding opportunities to continue juicing when you're traveling, that's a huge challenge. As soon as I got back home, I started right back on juicing again.

Shane: That's fantastic.

Nancy: You know, before I started my juice fast, I was already eating pretty healthy—mostly vegetables and limited poultry and fish. There wasn't a huge transition that some people have from eating hamburgers and fries and going right into juicing. One thing that I make that I really did miss was a gourmet veggie pizza with a fire-roasted crust, loaded with veggies and goat cheese. I honestly was craving that.

Shane: Nancy, the way you've just described that, I think everybody is going to be craving it.

Nancy: It is really good. But I just told myself, *It's not like you can never have this again. It's just right now that you need to focus on doing this juicing and then you can transition back to that.* I think that has prevented me from slipping up through my two juice fasts and saying to myself, "Don't stress. You're going to still get the opportunity to eat that again. It's just right now, this is what you're doing, your body needs to detox, and it's OK."

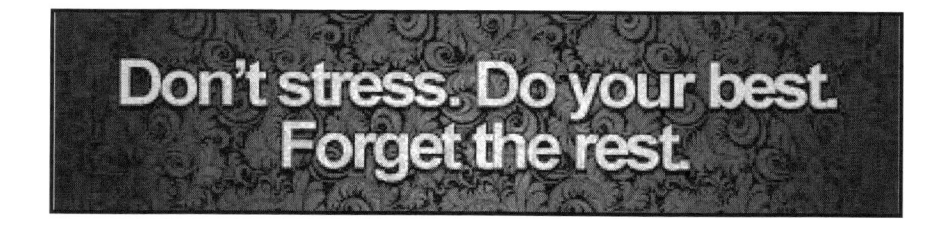

> Don't stress. Do your best. Forget the rest.

Shane: I love that strategy because I think you're absolutely right. If you're on a seven-day detox, or a 30-day detox, it's only one week or one month. The first few days are hard, but when you get to day four, you don't even think so much about food. That's the beauty.

You have to tell yourself, "It's not that I can never, ever have that apple pie again. I won't have it as much and I'll regulate it, and I'll make sure my diet is clean, but for the next week (or however long it might be), I can't have it." Even the word can't isn't quite right, as it's your choosing not to have it. You're saying "I can have it, but I don't want it."

Nancy: Right. So much is a choice and you're right, Shane. It is an absolute choice, and I think that for juicing, it's more than just a choice for seven days. It's a lifestyle choice, and it's something that you commit to. When I started, it wasn't that I was going to do this for seven days and be done. It was, "I'm going to do this for seven days and then I'm going to implement it in my transition and after my transition, where at least once a day I am juicing, if not twice a day, because I really enjoy the benefits from it." It's a long-term process. It's a long-term commitment. It's just simply a choice to have a new lifestyle.

Shane: It's fascinating to hear that because it's been four years ago since my first juice fast and I usually have several green juices a day, unless I've been traveling or on vacation. It has really become a part of my lifestyle rather than, "Oh, I have to detox. It's the first week of January, I have to detox." It's something I try to do every day. I'm at a stage where I miss my green juice if I don't get any. I really miss it.

Nancy: Right. It is great to see all the different juice bars popping up, and as a juicer, that gives me so many more options. I do love going to pick up a juice and then go for a long walk. It's just an integration into my lifestyle choice.

Shane: Nancy, did you receive any negative feedback from friends or family when you were on your juice fast?

Nancy: I kind of kept it a personal thing, so no, I didn't get any comments. Those who do know I'm juicing have been very supportive and I've appreciated that.

Shane: That's fantastic. What advice would you give to someone who's just starting a detox? What would you say to them based on the two fasts that you've completed and your weight loss success?

Nancy: I think that it's very important to have a multiple approach with your health and your well-being. To me, juicing is my daily infusion. When I drink the juice, I feel like I'm putting some really good things into my body, and it's this really healthy infusion. For me, it's not only doing the juicing, but it's also a daily infusion of mind, body, and spirit. I feel like that's why I have been so successful with my weight loss because it's been a multiple approach.

I also think that just as important as it is to juice and to eat very healthy, it's important to do things that mentally make you strong, that spiritually make you strong. I meditate, I pray, I do a lot of acts of service. That builds me up spiritually. Mind wise, I enjoy reading, for example, *The Charge,* is great and I enjoyed reading that.

Yes, I would encourage people to juice. It's life-altering, but also look at other aspects of your life, specifically the mind and spirit, and make it a body, mind, and spirit renewal, a reboot, whatever you want to call it. I think you will have more success because it's an overall approach that is really healthy and complete in creating a kind of wholeness in your perspective of life.

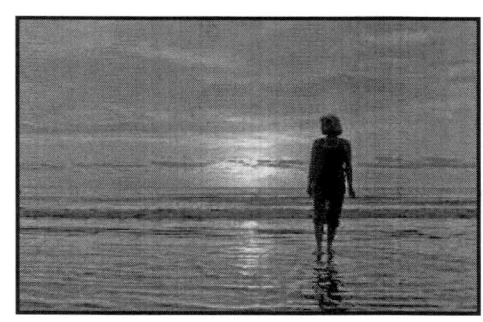

Shane: You mentioned *The Charge: Activating the 10 Human Drives That Make You Feel Alive* by Brendon Burchard. Is that relevant for juice detoxes?

Nancy: The book is all about feeling alive—different ideas and thoughts of feeling alive. If anything, juicing has made me feel alive. It's made me feel mentally strong, physically strong. It feels like an absolute daily infusion into my body that's brought me to a new level. So I would say that it's absolutely a good book, a good read, and there are definitely aspects that can apply to juicing in it.

Shane: Nancy, what habits did you create to really help you succeed on your first juice fast?

Nancy: One thing that I do is keep a calendar, weigh myself every day, and I record the weight. I also record goals that I have, but I keep little notes about how I did during the day with that juicing experience. I also keep a journal. Those two things are important to me, because I'm a very visual person. So to be able to see my progress in my journal or on the calendar is extremely important to me. I feel it contributes to my success in that process.

Shane: That's something that really means a lot to me. I urge everyone, when you go through your juice fasts, to journal daily. Each juice fast is very different, so you might juice fast really well on your first go, and on the second go, it might be a lot more difficult. Then you can read your notes of your first juice fast, particularly your notes from the first few days where generally you get the worst detox symptoms.

Then on day four you start writing about this crescendo of energy that you have, and you went for a run or you went swimming or you took the kids out and threw a ball around, whatever it might be. I think you can read all the self-help books in the world, all the inspirational themes, but when you read your own words—that's an absolute gold mine that you can tap into.

Nancy: I completely agree with that. One thing that was a little bit difficult, but it really helped me, was that I pulled out some old pictures of myself when I was at my heaviest weight. That was difficult, but at the same time it was very therapeutic. With juicing, one thing I've learned about the aspects of daily renewal is that it's absolutely never too late to take control of your life. It is all about being proactive, being your own advocate and really changing your life. Doing good things for your health, your mind, your spirit, and changing course.

You know, a lot of things happen in life, good and bad and everything in between. Ultimately, it's when you get to that point and you feel mentally, spiritually, and physically strong, you realize that you can't be conquered by those things. You can choose to be as strong as you want to be. You can absolutely have some really good things happen in your life and reach a level of happiness. That, for me, has been a long journey, but I'm only 15 pounds away from my goal, my final goal. I am so grateful for the journey and everything I've learned along the way.

Shane: Fantastic. We know you'll achieve your goal, and we're all excited for you!

Nancy: Thank you.

Shane: When you set that goal in the early days, it seems so far off. But you're on the cusp of achieving it. So I certainly congratulate you on your success.

Nancy: Thank you very much, Shane.

You can follow Nancy
and her amazing plant-based recipes at
https://twitter.com/APPETITEology

Get your free copy of
How to Get Started with Juicing
and receive free email juice coaching
(but not spam—that's not healthy).

Sign up at www.juicinghabits.com

JUICING RADIO

Shane and Angie invite you to listen to a juicing success story every week on Juicing Radio.

Sign up for updates and never miss an episode at JuicingRadio.com.

So Inspirational

by MariBrian

I look forward each week to this podcast. There is so much information packed into an hour. The best thing is the interviews with "real" people like you and me. And Shane and Angie are so relatable. I feel like we're all sitting around my kitchen talking whenever I listen to it.

Chapter 7
Shawny
Affirms Her Process to Health

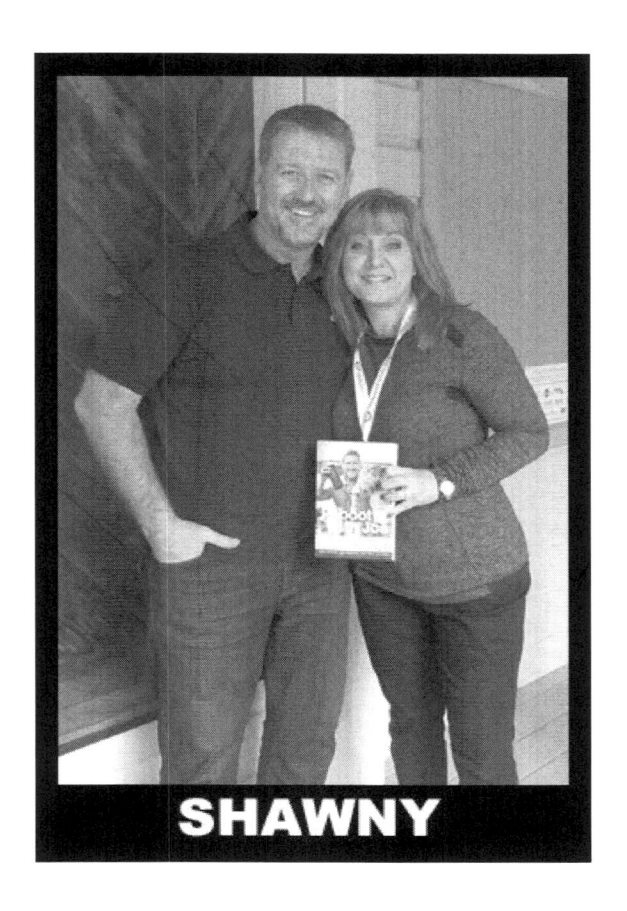

SHAWNY

Angie: Juicing Radio followed Shawny during her 30-day juice fast. That's right; she was able to complete a 30-day reboot on juice only. Hi, Shawny! Where are you from?

Shawny: Hi, Angie. I'm from Ottawa, Canada.

Angie: You've been on the Juicing Radio podcasts quite a few times and you're also on the Camp Reboot panel.

Shawny: That's correct. I loved it. It was great to be there and finally meet you in person.

Angie: What made you start juicing or start a juice fast?

Shawny: Over the years, like many people, I've tried all kinds of diets. Battling weight has been the story of my life and I was always looking for that magical diet or food regimen that would get me to where I wanted to be. I tried all the big names. I went to all the meetings. I have a host of diet books, more than I can count, in my library. I watched *Fat, Sick and Nearly Dead* and within a few days, I went out and bought a juicer. That's pretty much how I got hooked on juicing. It was *Fat, Sick and Nearly Dead* and the transformation that Joe Cross went through. It was just so inspiring to me and it seemed like a really helpful, sane way of going about weight loss and getting back your health.

Angie: Well, you're not alone there. I don't know how many people I've heard say, "I watched the movie and then I went out and bought the juicer and started." What program did you follow or did you follow a program?

Shawny: I really didn't follow a program, per se. I went online and discovered some juice recipes, a website where I was able to discover some great tips and tricks about what to juice and what might go together. I am a bit of a gourmet cook on the side. I've always been passionate about cooking, and I'm pretty good with knowing what flavors go together. I really enjoyed sort of freestyle juicing. In the beginning, I did the Mean Green and I used a lot of fruit to sweeten the juice until my palate was ready for the more robust type of juices. Basically it was really freestyle juicing for me.

Angie: Let's go back to what you said about doing a lot of Mean Green and you also did a lot of more fruit-heavy juices. For people who might not have done a juice fast before, what do you mean by that? What do you mean by changing your palate?

Shawny: When you jump into juicing, sometimes the more heavily based leafy-green juices are a little tougher to get used to. Seasoned juicers can attest to that, especially if you're juicing greens like kale. I'd never even heard of kale before I started juicing. I had no idea what it was. All I knew was that kale was this huge, rubbery, giant, leafy-green vegetable and it took up half the grocery cart. I didn't know what it tasted like and sometimes I'd put too much in the juice. I thought, the recipe calls for three leaves of kale, but I was freestyling. I thought, *Well kale is good for me, so I'll put six or seven leaves in,* not knowing what it was going to taste like. It was a bit of a chemistry experiment in the beginning.

By adding more pineapple or lemon or orange to cut the taste, I was able to get the green juice down a lot easier. As you progress through juicing, you'll find that you wean yourself off the sweetness. Now I go with more of an 80/20 kind of ratio—80 percent veggie and 20 percent fruit in my juices, just to kind of have a little bit of sweet but not too much.

Angie: I find that most people have to work up to the 80/20. Most people can't start out that way. When you're starting something new, it's so important to make sure your first experiences are positive, because you tend to have a negative association if you drink something that's really off your palate. You might not try it again, so in the beginning it's important to use fruits and vegetables that you know you like. I had a rule that if I didn't like it, I would just add another apple.

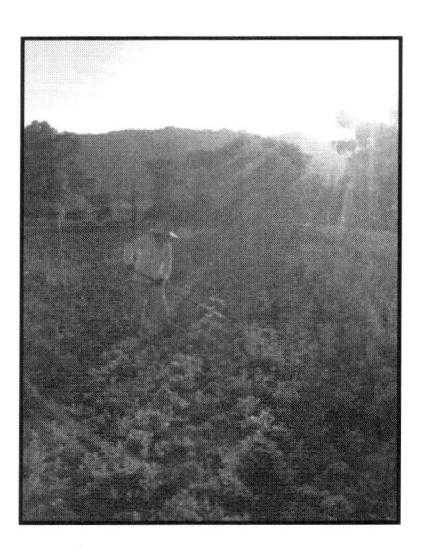

Shawny: Oh, there you go. That's good.

Angie: This kind of experimentation is good because everybody's palate is different and can tolerate different ratios. I've heard from a lot of our highly successful juicers who didn't follow a program. They did what you did—freestyling. Everyone is starting in a different place and it's a good idea to experiment and find what works for you.

Shawny: Absolutely, and it's a lot of fun too, because you really feel like you're building up to something and you don't know how it's going to turn out. I don't think I've ever had two juices that tasted exactly the same. There's always something a little different about them, you know? One of the things I found that helps is adding spices, such as Tabasco sauce or pepper. At Camp Reboot we added turmeric, cinnamon, or nutmeg to juices and that's another great way to have them taste a little better, especially in the beginning if you're not too sure about the taste. You can always add some spice or herbs to give it a whole new dimension, a whole new flavor.

Angie: That's a really good tip. I love spicy juices. That's a great way to positively enhance some flavors that you might not be so thrilled about. A lot of people express being really scared to start a juice fast. Were you scared at all or did you have any fears, and, if so, how did you cope with that?

Shawny: You know, I don't think I was scared at all. I was really excited to actually start it because I had seen Joe's movie and his results. I thought, *Surely if it worked for him, it's going to work for me.* I was just so impressed with him and he also seemed so healthy. He wasn't counting calories, and didn't have to go to meetings and say how he did all week. He was just doing his own thing and that really appealed to me, because perhaps I'm a bit of a lone wolf. I like doing my own thing and I wasn't scared at all to embark on this journey. I really felt like there was something that ignited in me when I watched that movie. There was a spark and I knew that if I tried this, it was going to work.

Angie: The big inspirational spark is a major turning point for a lot of people. Why else do you think that your juice fasts have been successful? What kinds of habits have you developed?

Shawny: When I went out and bought the juicer and came home with it and unpacked it, I had already cleared a spot on my counter, dedicated for it in my kitchen. I'm a person who's very organized and tidy, and I don't have much on my countertops. But this juicer was going to have its very own place.

Angie: Wow, a place of honor.

Shawny: Absolutely, because I knew if I didn't make provisions to have a special place for it to reside, it wasn't going to be used. That was important to me to have a dedicated spot.

The other thing I did was to stock up on Mason jars, because you've got to have containers to put the juice in once you've prepared it. One of the funny, important things I do with my Mason jars, to give me inspiration on a daily basis, is I write myself little messages on the lids. So when I pull one out to drink it, it'll say something like "Juice on" or things that Joe said. I'll write with a Sharpie pen on the containers, "You can do it" or "Just juice it" and put smiley faces on them. It gives me that extra little sort of cheer.

Angie: I love that. The juice affirmations.

Shawny: There you go, juice affirmations.

Angie: I also love what you said about putting your juicer out on the counter, because the best juicer is the one you're actually going to use. If it's not out and convenient then it lowers the odds that you're actually going to do it. Those are great tips.

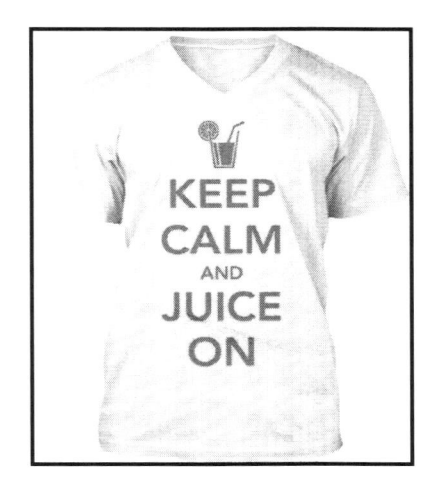

Shawny: Thanks.

Angie: I know you've done quite a few juice fasts. I think your first juice fast was about 18 days and then you did a 30-day juice fast. From either one of those experiences do you remember having an "aha" moment or when things really clicked and you had a deeper understanding of how to move forward?

Shawny: I think the biggest "aha" for me was just coming to the realization that this was actually working. I could actually sustain myself on juice, on liquid alone. I was amazed. I thought, *Oh, my gosh, a liquid fast. How am I going to do that? How I am going to get through that? Surely I'm going to be depleted of energy. I'm going to be hungry. I'm going to be cranky.* I did go through some hungry and cranky spots, but for the most part, I was blown away by the energy I had. Once you experience that, it's just the best natural high. It really is and you think, *Wow, I've got so much energy. I don't need as much sleep because I'm sleeping better.* My "aha" moment was thinking, *Wow, this stuff really works and I'm going to stick with this.* I was so happy about how I was actually feeling.

Angie: What was your biggest challenge?

Shawny: One of the challenges for me was the preparation of the juice. That's tough when you're working fulltime and you've got a family that counts on you to prepare their food. Juicing can take a lot of time, so it took me a while to tweak it. I would basically juice at night and then prepare everything for the next day. That worked for a while. Then there were evenings when I was too tired, so I'd have to get up early the next morning and do it. Juicing at 5:00 a.m. really doesn't work.

Angie: That's pretty early.

Shawny: Yeah, it's just not great. What I like to do now is take a few hours on a Sunday afternoon and prepare all my juice for the week and freeze it. That works really well for me right now. I'll juice about 30 to 35 Mason jars of juice, and I don't fill them to the top because I don't want them to explode or crack in the freezer.

Angie: Right.

Shawny: I've had that happen to me and it was a lesson learned. So my jars are lined up like little soldiers in the freezer, and I take them out the night before and pop them into my lunch bag that I have for work and take them with me. It's fantastic. They taste delicious and then I have my nights free, which is great, to do things with my family.

Angie: That's a great time-saving tip. Gosh, how long does it take you to do 30 juices?

Shawny: I'd say anywhere from three-and-a-half to four-and-a-half hours.

Angie: That's a significant time commitment, but if you're preparing juice every day, you would probably spend more time than that because you have to clean the juicer each time.

Shawny: Exactly. It's a lot of work but for me this really seems to be working right now. I think it's a great time saver for me during the week. I do the preparation of the veggies on the weekends. I'll fill the sink with water and let them soak. I've got one specific juice that I do at a time and then I move on to the next juice. Then I clean the juicer in between. I actually have two juicers going—one is a slow juicer and I've got another juicer that works well on the harder vegetables, such as carrots and beets. It's like a big juice fest on Sunday afternoon.

Angie: You've got a full production going on.

Shawny: I do.

Angie: You said that one of your challenges was finding the time and even though it wasn't completely easy in the beginning, you did mornings and evenings and then eventually you came to the conclusion that you're a weekend juicer.

Shawny: Yes.

Angie: You were also cooking for your family while you were juice fasting, correct?

Shawny: Yes, and I don't know how I did that. There were some nights I was up until 11:00 p.m. juicing. I'd get home from work, make their dinner, clean up, and then next thing I know, I've got to get these juices prepped for the next day. In the beginning, I prepared juice for one day and then I got wise and I juiced two to three days. Now I'm at the point where I juice for a week and freeze everything. It's just easier for me.

Angie: Wow, you are a very determined lady.

Shawny: Very, but that's kind of my personality. Once you say go, it's full throttle!

Angie: So when you were cooking or when you weren't cooking, did you have any specific cravings during your juice fast and how did you overcome those?

Shawny: I would walk into the supermarket and smell things. I was cooking, so of course I had cravings. When I smelled things I wanted, I'd make sure I always had juice or water or gum nearby. I chewed a lot of gum. I think that's the sensation you miss the most is the chewing. And when you smell something cooking, it conjures up memories of eating and chewing, so the gum was really my best friend—feeling like I was consuming something, but I wasn't.

That got me over the hump. The cravings really subsided after I'd say maybe five days. Then you really don't crave anything anymore. You're starting to see results at that point and you've come through the fog, come through the first three days that are a little more challenging. You don't have headaches anymore. You're not running to the bathroom all the time. You've come through it OK at that point and then the cravings do subside, definitely.

The other thing I did was preparing myself before the fast. I've been a vegan now for a year so I eat fairly well, but when I did my first juice fast I read up on what I needed to do and it was important to go to a basic, clean diet. If you can, try to eliminate dairy, meats, sugar, alcohol, and coffee leading up to the fast, just to prepare your body and get things going so that when you go to all juice it's really quite seamless. The detox is a lot less harsh.

Angie: When you stay the detox is less harsh, what do you mean exactly? Please explain it for people who don't know.

Shawny: What I mean is that you don't have as much to eliminate from your body because when you're doing just juice, especially the first three days, your body just absorbs the juice and starts to clean you out. It's the detox and you're getting rid of a lot of impurities in your body. Another part of detox is the headaches that come from caffeine withdrawal. So if you can help prepare your body, if you can do that, good for you. My first juice fast I did not give up coffee, because I just thought it's my only vice. Cut me some slack.

Angie: You're perfect in every way, Shawny.

Shawny: Except for the coffee. I'm not quite there, but I'm trying. Then my second juice fast, I actually did eliminate the coffee and that was a little harder on my system, but definitely worthwhile. I think it also made a difference about how the fast went.

Angie: Well, there are a few things you just said that I really love. One is prepping yourself before a juice fast—really being ready for it. The more you prepare, the easier the actual juice fast will be.

Shawny: Definitely.

Angie: I also love that you kind of met yourself halfway on your first juice fast and you knew that it would be really difficult for you to give up coffee. Instead of saying, "Well, then, I'm just not going to do it, because I just can't give up my coffee," you actually went ahead and did a juice fast and modified it.

Shawny: Yes.

Angie: And guess what? On your next juice fast, you did a little better—a lot better!

Shawny: That's right.

Angie: You gave up coffee completely and you did 30 days the second time.

Shawny: That's right, versus 18 days the first time. It was definitely a success story the second time around. I don't think that the first one wasn't a success story because I learned a lot. I learned what my body could tolerate and what juices worked for me and which ones didn't and eventually why I had to throw in the towel on that one at day 18. When I took on the 30-day challenge, I already was armed with the information I had from that first juice fast and I was a lot more successful.

Angie: What I love is that you just went forward, and did your best. At least you tried the first time and then the next time you did a little better.

Shawny: That's true. I think sometimes we're just too hard on ourselves and that's why we fall down and we're not successful. If you don't think you can give something up, like the coffee, then don't give it up that first time. Just do your best. If it's the only thing that's your crutch, then that's OK. At least you've eliminated everything else. I think you have to listen to your body and know what your limitations are. Then you know the next time you can push forward a little more and try something even a little riskier.

Angie: Right, and everybody starts at a different place. Not everyone will be able to do several days on juice only and some people might start with one juice a day for a while and then work up to doing more days. I like what you said about being gentle with yourself and not being too hard on yourself, because no major change comes out of a place of shame. If you're feeling shamed, your mindset isn't right. You don't have the right mental juice yet.

Shawny: You're absolutely correct, Angie. That is an awesome quote. I love that.

Angie: Did you have any negative feedback when you were juice fasting, and, if so, how did you cope with that?

Shawny: I didn't really have a lot of negative feedback. People expected that I would research healthy things and try new ideas. I think they wanted to actually see me do it and succeed. I would explain to them what I was doing and they were really intrigued by it and very encouraging. I'm lucky that I'm surrounded by a positive support team in my family, and my colleagues are incredible. The folks I work with are just amazing and during the past couple of years, I'd say about 10 people in my office now have juicers and juice.

Angie: Wow, you've really influenced a lot of people.

Shawny: I have, and it's really a lot of fun. We talk juice at work daily. We compare our juices. We line them up on the cubicle desks and we look at the colors and we smell one another's juices.

Angie: You've created your own little juicing tribe.

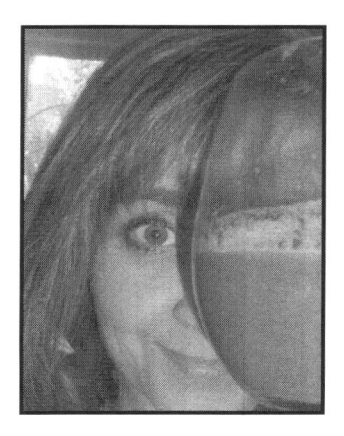

Shawny: I have!

Angie: I think it's good to create your own tribe. You become the role model and then people will gravitate toward you if they are interested. You gain strength and support from one another.

One other thing you said was that you explained what you were doing and why you were doing it. That's a great idea if you sit down with your family and friends and share with them.

Shawny: Definitely, yes.

Angie: If you can have a real authentic conversation about why juicing is important to you and ask them for their support, then you're much more likely to have understanding folks around you. Sometimes the hardest thing to do is to ask people for help or to ask people for support, but you know these people care about you. If they know something is really important to you, my guess is that most people will be supportive.

Shawny: Definitely. You're right about that because my family has seen me try every diet on the planet so they might have been a little skeptical in the beginning when I brought home yet another small appliance. But they watched the movie with me, so they knew what it was all about. They had seen the success, so they were very encouraging for me to try this.

I'm one of the lucky people, and you're absolutely right about having support. Let's face it, a lot of us have exhausted all kinds of other avenues in this effort to get healthy and change our lives. We try a new diet that we hope is going to be the key this time. When you've tried everything else and you're turning to this, some people do think it's a gimmick. If you sit down and are honest with them and tell them how much this means to you to have their support, I don't think there are too many families that would not support you.

Angie: Well, you've given so many great tips for new juicers. Is there any advice that you would give to somebody who's starting their first juice fast?

Shawny: I'd say to definitely take your time in selecting a juicer that's right for you. Do your homework. There's a lot of information online that you can access.

And be sure that you make juices that you know you're going to enjoy the taste of. That's really important. If you don't like it, you're definitely not going to drink it. And you have to make sure you consume at least 64 to 96 ounces of juice a day on a juice fast. Be sure that you like what you're making.

Another tip is I like to buy frozen berries. I'll buy bags of frozen berries when they're on sale, and later I'll thaw them in the fridge and juice them. That's one way to save money, because produce can be expensive.

Angie: Yes, that's a good tip. Are there any other habits that helped you succeed with your first juice fast or any of your subsequent juice fasts?

Shawny: One of the things I really like to do is journal. I go to a good bookshop and buy a nice-looking journal. I like to copy inspirational quotes in my journal, and every day I write what I'm consuming in juice and how much water or coconut water I'm taking in and the activities that I've done during the day. I also record my mood and other things.

When you're juice fasting, you go through a lot of different transformations along the way as you progress. Especially if you're on it for 30 days, one week to the next can be quite different. So I like to record that and then I like to look back and see the progress along the way and how I was feeling. I even keep recipes in the journal of some concoctions that I've made and tested that were delicious, so I don't forget how to make them. An important thing for me is journaling, for sure.

Angie: That's another great tip, Shawny. You are truly a highly successful juicer. Thank you so much for sharing your habits.

Shawny: Thank you for what you do! One of the reasons for my success has definitely involved social media and connecting with other juicers either through Juicing Radio or through the Reboot with Joe website. It's really great to know that you have support and that you have juicing friends who can be there when you're having a tough day or give you advice on things or share recipes. So thank you very much for what you do. It's been great.

Angie: You're very welcome. Here's to juicing friends.

Shawny's Favorite Links for Vegan, Gluten Free, and Juicing Recipes

http://ohsheglows.com/
http://glutenfreegoddess.blogspot.ca/
http://www.veganricha.com/
https://www.youtube.com/user/FullyRawKristina
http://engine2diet.com/
https://juicerecipes.com/recipes/ (great for recipes with ingredients you have on-hand)

Shawny's Favorite Juicing Recipes for Late Summer

Watermelon, lime, and mint—so very refreshing!

I also enjoy plum, peach, and nectarine, as the fruit is delicious this time of year! The juice is little thicker—almost like a nectar—but, oh, so yummy!

Get your free copy of
How to Get Started with Juicing
**and receive free email juice coaching
(but not spam—that's not healthy).**

Sign up at www.juicinghabits.com

JUICING RADIO

Shane and Angie invite you to listen to a juicing success story every week on Juicing Radio.

Sign up for updates and never miss an episode at
JuicingRadio.com.

Great Shows, Great People!!

by Abeautifulmess

I was so honored to share my story with juicing radio. Shane and Angie do a fantastic job every week and I have tried recipes from What Juicers Eat and they were all fantastic!! Keep up the great work!!

Shane's 7 Keys to Successful Juicing Weight Loss

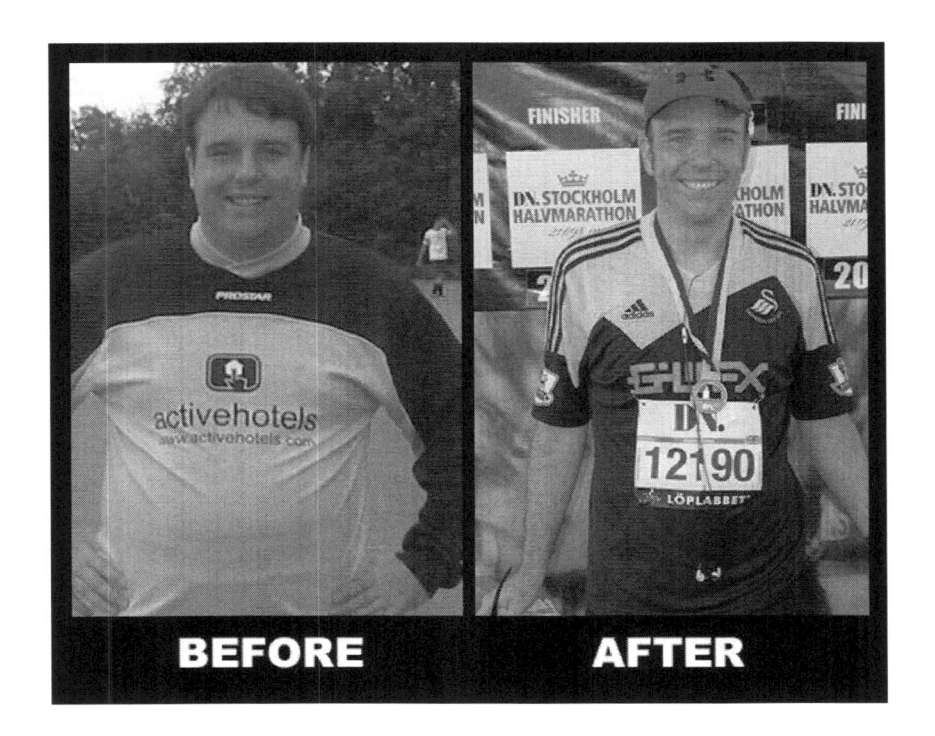

BEFORE **AFTER**

Introduction

Are you interested in juicing but never tried? Are you in the middle of the juice fast, or just about to transition to a balanced diet? Whatever the stage, this bonus chapter is for you. It includes useful tips and resources, inspiring and empowering you to change your life for good.

The seven keys to successful juicing in this chapter are from someone who has been where you are, he's an ordinary guy who managed to lose 80 pounds while running on juice. He's juice fanatic Shane Whaley. He shared these ideas as a response to some listener questions on the Juicing Radio podcast.

People follow Shane's story and have a lot of questions. Many of those questions center on how he started and why he was successful; how he went from an overweight guy with no energy and poor skin, to drop 80 pounds. Here's what he has to share.

The Early Part of My Journey

I went back over my notes, and it was surprising how many I'd kept from the early part of my journey. I figured what I would do is try to distill some of the success into seven keys to my successful juicing. My juice fast, the first one I ever did, was seven days. It was in January 2010. I was very overweight. I had a high-stress job. I had no energy. My eating habits were poor. I certainly did not exercise in any way, shape, or form, unless it was running to the bar for last orders.

So I went back over my notes, and I've distilled them to seven keys that I really want to share, because this is a really large serving of "mental juice." I hope it inspires you, particularly if you're at the start of your journey or if you've fallen off the wagon, so to say. Maybe you're just back from vacation, and you've put on those pounds and think, "Right. Now is the time I'm going to sort my health out."

You might know about my "aha" moments, both in business and in personal, when that lady poked me in my stomach in the middle of a bar, telling me I needed to lose weight—always nice when that happens. So now, I want to talk about the seven keys.

First Key—Scribe

It's essential that you've got all the juice ingredients, you know what recipes you're going to make, and you're set. It's either the evening before or the morning of your first juice fast. What's really important is to write down your hopes and aspirations. Why do you want to juice? Why do you want to get healthy?

It's really important you know that before you even set off. There's an old quote, I believe by business author Brian Tracy, that says, "If it's to be, it's up to me." You can't rely on anyone else here. You can get all the inspiration you want, but your mind has got to be in the right gear to be able to complete your first juicing, whether it's a cleanse or you're just incorporating lots more juice into your life. It's so important that you're driven on this, and you need to find your waypoint.

Once you do that, then write down the plan of how you intend getting there. In my case, I knew that I had to go through a seven-day Jason Vale, Juicemaster.com, juice plan. Remember, this was before Reboot with Joe. This was before *Fat, Sick and Nearly Dead.* There was very little information out there, certainly not as much as there is now.

I love the fact that now there are tons of blogs and Facebook pages and YouTube channels. I remember, in my early days when I was feeling "hungry," going online and desperately searching for juicing success stories because I needed that inspiration. Although my mind was in full throttle toward the goal, I wanted some reassurance. In early 2010, there wasn't that much online about juicing, only some hippie recipes. No offense, but I'm sure you know what I mean.

I recently pulled out my old notebook, and it's really emotional to read some of the notes, because I made them about my health, about my career. I'll share something that's not related to juicing but just shows you how powerful this is. In 2010, I wrote, "I want to be the area manager for my company in the United States."

At the time, I was a Brit living in Stockholm, Sweden, and my dream had always been to live and work in the United States. I know there's a lot of debate about immigration right now, but basically back then there was no way I was ever going to get a green card or a visa. I tried in the 1990s, and the US government basically said, "You're a sales guy. You're a good sales guy, but we don't need more sales guys. You need some real specialist skills to get in."

But I wrote this as one of my goals. I now live in New York City. I spent three years in San Francisco—three great years in California. I'm just celebrating my second anniversary of living in Manhattan. I really don't think it would have happened if I hadn't set the goals for myself. It was also very, very important to sort my health out.

It was no coincidence that my career rocketed at the Fortune 500 company I was working with, once I sorted out my health. I think that's because of two things. First, clearly, I had a lot more energy. When you start dropping the weight, when you start exercising, it gives you that mental clarity. It sharpens your focus, and I strongly believe I was able to achieve better business results. I certainly know I was a better manager of people because I had a lot more energy and drive.

The second thing, a little controversial, is I really feel that certain people in the organization saw I dropped the weight. I think there is a perception that many of us who are overweight, maybe we're lazy, which is completely untrue for most of us, but there is that perception. So I really feel that my business results spoke for themselves, but it was also my improved appearance, and that is why I was given the opportunity—my dream move to transfer from Stockholm to San Francisco for a great promotion, by the way. It wasn't just a sideways move. This was a really good promotion.

So write down your hopes and your aspirations. I wrote my career goals, and I wrote my health goals. I actually wrote in the present tense, "I am loving being 85 kilos." I was living in Europe then, and 85 kilos is about 188 pounds. At this time, I weigh about 177. So I'm actually 10 pounds less than I was forecasting. My original goal was 70 pounds or so of weight loss. So I was able to overachieve, and I strongly believe it was because I wrote down my goals. I had my why-power of what I wanted to do.

Something I'm going to point out is that January in Sweden is really bloody cold. It was about negative 30 Fahrenheit and about three feet of snow. I juiced through that first week in really freezing temperatures.

After you write your goal, you need to write down a plan of how you intend to get to your goal. So I'd written my goal that I wanted to complete in seven days. I wanted to clean up my eating. I wanted to take some cooking classes (I never actually did that, but it was written down). I wanted to exercise some more.

What I did was establish a baseline of where I was. So I knew I wasn't going to go out and train for a marathon. I mean, you're talking about a guy who couldn't even run for five minutes. So I established a baseline. I set a goal. Then I defined a clear path toward that goal.

I made it, and those of you who work in business have probably heard this before, but I made it a smart goal. So it was specific. It was measurable. It was attainable. It was realistic, and it was time-based, which is something I use in my job, because you have to have a realistic goal.

I did say I wanted to drop 70 pounds, but then I said, "Okay. In two months, I want to drop X amount." On my exercise goals, I actually wrote that I wanted to be able to run 30 minutes nonstop. That was my goal. There was none of this half-marathon, marathon, run 1,000 miles a year, whatever else, a Spartan race. It was, "I want to be able to run nonstop for 30 minutes."

Even though I went on from that initial goal to run four half-marathons and thousands of miles in training, I still say to people that my proudest achievement in my weight loss and in changing my health was that first time I ever ran 30 minutes nonstop, because at that stage, it might as well have been a marathon. When I was on that first week of making my plan, I dreamed of running 30 minutes nonstop. I thought it would be really hard work, and it *was* hard work.

I think the difference is when you get to those 30 minutes, you then have confidence to push on. Then you start to say, "Okay. I want to run 10K now," because you know you've got that base fitness to where you can run for 30 minutes.

Keep a journal of successes, struggles, and humbling moments during your juicing. So I've got all mine written in front of me. As I say, it was quite emotional to look back at my notes. But I'd write down at the end of the day how I didn't go and buy a burger at lunchtime, or go and have a pint of beer after work. I would write about how I was feeling. I felt it was very useful for me to do that because I'd read that every day. I'd read the previous day's entry, and it just gives you something really to build on.

So that's your first key. I call it scribe. Write your goals and your plans down.

Second Key—Sharing

I strongly believe to increase your chances of success, share your plan. Share your goal, whether it be with family or with friends. You have to commit, and commit publicly. I felt that was a great help to me. I didn't want to be a secret juicer. I wanted everyone to know, so that they wouldn't put a hot dog in front of me, or if I was a little bit cranky, or if I wasn't going down to the pub to watch the football, they knew why.

Also, at that stage, bear in mind, it was 2010. Juicing wasn't as popular as it is now. And a lot of people would say, "Yeah, you'll never do that. You'll never do juice-only for seven days." That actually spurred me on to prove them wrong.

The other thing I did (and with social media today, this is much easier to utilize) was to set up a blog. Some of you might be familiar with it; it's called RunningOnJuice.com. Now, I don't really update that blog anymore because the podcast takes a lot of time, but back then I started blogging.

I started writing about what juice I was drinking, how I was feeling, how to make the juice, how to clean up, what my running was like. That blog got a really good following and some people have been reading it me since the Running on Juice days. That was a great help, because I felt I was being held accountable because all these people were coming to the blog and commenting. I didn't want to let them down.

Even fairly recently, I tested out the Jason Vale Five Pounds in Five Days program. I podcast every day during that program about my success and my journey and how it was going and my thoughts and tactics and strategies. Even though I consider myself an experienced juicer, that still held me accountable. I still knew when I had my weak moments that, "Oh, so what am I going to say on the podcast tomorrow? Well, you know what? They're having pizza in the office or cupcakes, and I ate one. I'm sorry."

I wanted to do this for two reasons. First, I wanted to keep everyone engaged, and I didn't want to let anyone down. But also, I really wanted to test the Five Pounds in Five Days program because I never recommend anything unless I've tried it. I wanted to see what the results were like, but more important I wanted to know how I felt on that particular plan.

So set up a Facebook account, if you haven't already, a Twitter feed, Google Plus, and Pinterest. I mean, there are so many different ways of doing it, but sharing your journey and what you're doing will hold you accountable. All these supports can be the winning edge. In fact, when you're at a low point, and you're feeling "hungry," or you want to give up, or you're feeling tired, low on energy. You say, "Well, what am I going to say to everyone tomorrow? I failed." Nobody wants to write that.

Third Key—Reach Out

There is now a plethora of resources online that you can utilize. So join online communities, such as RebootwithJoe.com. It has a very thriving forum. If you join the group, you'll make a lot of online friends. You get to read about other people's journeys, other people's successes, their tips, and nice recipes. It's really important that you lock into the Reboot with Joe community. I'm not being paid to say that. I am an ambassador for Joe Cross, but I don't receive any money for that. I would have loved that community when I was starting out in 2010. It would have been a huge help.

Then on top of that, there are so many great Facebook groups. I recommend Juicing for Dummies, run by Leslie and Trace Justice. That's a phenomenal group, very active, with a lot of great people who will help you, whether you're at a low moment or you need some reassurance, or you want some help with a recipe or picking out a juicer, or just a bit of inspiration. There are a lot of before-and-after photos on there. So I would definitely join Juicing for Dummies.

There's another great group in Canada, Juicing 101. There are groups in the United Kingdom. You can join the community and you don't even have to post. Just reading all the comments will really help you.

Of course, there is Juicing Radio, at least once a week. All the back episodes are available to listen to for hours of juicing content. I know I'm blowing my own horn here a little bit, but that's an amazing resource, and particularly because we interview successful juicers. In episode one, there was an interview with Brian Robertson, who lost 165 pounds and many of his multiple sclerosis (MS) symptoms decreased. And there was an interview with Amy Beard, who dropped 66 pounds by doing a 90-day cleanse, even while working as a diner chef.

Again, I would have loved to have had these resources when I started out. I used to really desperately search the Internet, looking for any success story I could to help me get through the day. So use Juicing Radio by going to the archives and listening to past shows. There are also Juicing Radio shows on iTunes. These will help keep you inspired, to give you a big fresh serving of mental juice. Of course, there are movies you can watch. So check out the websites, Facebook pages, Twitter, etc.

So that's key number three—reach out. So far, we've had key number one—scribe, key number two—to share, and key number three to successful juicing—reach out.

Fourth Key—Cut the Distractions

This is a difficult one; I have to be honest. When I was on my first juice-only, I was a single guy. I didn't have to cook for a loved one. I didn't have kids. So I was able to do it myself. If you do have family, maybe try to get your partner to cook for the family that first week or come up with other arrangements.

I know it's really tough, but then I hear stories like Amy, who was flipping burgers all day in a diner and was still able to juice. So it is possible, and that's all about having the right why-power. That's a really good podcast for people to listen to when they're starting out.

I remember one juice fast I was on when I was in San Francisco. I was flicking through Netflix and I ended up watching, subconsciously, *Man v. Food.* About five minutes in, I'm like, "Why am I torturing myself here? Why am I doing this to myself?" And it reminded me of the time I gave up cigarettes—awful, disgusting, dirty habit. I remember I gave up cold turkey, from 40 a day to none. It was weird. Every time I turned the TV on, I wouldn't even notice what the characters were saying. I'd be like, "Oh, he's smoking a cigarette. That looks good. James Bond is smoking a cigar. I want a cigar."

It's the same as when I'm rebooting. You hone in on what people are eating. It is a form of torture, especially if it's your first juicing experience. So be very careful about that. The other thing is don't walk past your favorite restaurants. I live in lower Manhattan and when I took my dog for her 20-minute walk, I counted 27 food places. That can be torture. So I have to take a different route because I'm only human.

The waft of an Indian meal or pizza or whatever else tempts you, on the early days of a juice fast, can be the thing that will topple you over the edge. And the smell of fish and chips is one of the strongest compelling marketing ploys a business can have. So try not to walk past your favorite restaurants. Don't read cookbooks. Don't read magazines that you subscribe to which are food-based. Yeah, cut that out.

If you can, and I know this isn't always possible, clear your social diary for that week. If you've got a party or a business event, that can be hard just because you see food being served, and then you've got the pressure of explaining to people, "No, I'm on a juice cleanse." That's really tough, because people don't get it. Then they start talking to you about it.

It's like when you go for dinner, and you've had a really nice meal, and someone says, "Oh, they have really good cheesecake here." Now, you have no intention of having the cheesecake, but they do, and they feel better if you also have that cheesecake. So you have to really watch out when you're at some social events.

So that's number four—cut the distractions. I posted about this, that I was on day three of my last reboot and I got the dog her food, but she wouldn't eat it. I'm looking at this dog food, and it just smelled great. Right? How embarrassing that I'm looking at the dog's food, because it's day three on a juice fast. So even the dog food had me thinking about food, and it's disgusting stuff.

Fifth Key—Train Your Brain

I think this is crucial. Well, they're all crucial, but this one in particular is what saved me. I'm going to call it, "Train Your Brain." So the important thing to do here, during your juice-only fast, if possible, is watching as many inspirational documentaries as you can during that period. *Fat, Sick and Nearly Dead* is compulsory viewing. I've seen that film many times, but every time I do a reboot, I watch it.

Here's my tip. It's really important that you buy the DVD. This is why. I believe the DVD has more than 90 minutes of additional content. Joe Cross shot about 500-plus hours of footage for that movie, and he had to condense it to an hour and a half. So there are a lot of stories, a lot of interviews that he couldn't put into the movie.

So what I would do is, say I'm starting my fast on a Monday, I would either watch the whole movie that night, or I'd break it in half so I have something to watch the following night. Then I would go through the extras and the bonus content. I would watch as many of the interviews as I could that were cut from the movie, and then the next thing I would do is watch the movie again but with the director's commentary. So Joe actually talks you through the movie. There's a lot of stuff he talks about in the commentary that isn't in the film, which I find really important in terms of training the brain.

Jason Vale has a fantastic movie out, *Super Juice Me.* This is just what you want to see when you're on a juice fast. There's also *Powered by Green Smoothies.* You have to be a little bit careful, because there are great documentaries, such as *Food, Inc.,* and *Hungry for Change.* But I found if I watch those too early in the juice fast—because they talk about food—my mind is going on and on about food. So I would tend to wait until day four for those documentaries. I would keep the first couple of nights for juice-only, and then I would watch *Forks over Knifes* and similar movies after the first few nights.

Read inspirational books. They don't necessarily have to be about juicing. It could be one of your political heroes, or a film star who you follow, or a pop singer. I mean, I love Morrissey, though I'm not sure I'd read his autobiography when I'm on a juice fast because I don't know how uplifting that is. But try and read some books and use that time in the evening when you would normally be cooking or watching a movie. Get a book from the library that you've been meaning to read for ages. That will help you.

Toward the end of your fast, start picking up some books on nutrition, so you know how to transition out and how you want to eat after your reboot. Angie, my partner at Juicing Radio, covers this a lot on What Juicers Eat. If you're not on it already, please sign up to get her emails every week.

The basis behind that is that Angie dropped 86 pounds through juicing, cleaner eating, and running. She'd never run before either, by the way, until she started juicing. So we kept hearing from people who said, "What should I eat post-juicing?" Angie shares one of her recipes that she's discovered and sends it out free of charge. If you go to Whatjuicerseat.com, it's a very easy signup process, and you can get those emails in your inbox.

Another thing you can do is watch *Food Matters*, which is a lot of these documentaries. You can browse through there and it's really good to watch during your fast and afterward. There's a lot of inspirational stuff and it's encouraging to have that service.

As part of Train Your Brain, what's extremely important is visualization. A lot of top athletes and film stars use this technique. When I first heard about visualization, I thought it was all part of that woo-woo stuff and didn't really work. If I sit there and visualize myself as a millionaire, suddenly I'm going to become a millionaire.

But I'll tell you something now, and I'm looking at my notes. I was visualizing myself slimmer, leaner, more energy. I even wrote down, "When I lose the weight, I can play football again." That's soccer, for Americans. "I can be a referee. I want to run a half-marathon." So there were a lot of things that I would visualize.

I was looking through some other notes in my notebook and found that people often asked me, "So you started juicing in the extreme winter in Scandinavia. How on Earth did you go outside and run and juice?" Actually, what I would do is I would step out the door. After the initial shock of it being negative 30, I used to have 10 reasons in my head of why I was doing this. I'll quickly run through them because, again, this is really important for your successful juicing. You might be able to think of 10 reasons why you're juicing. Have those in your mind. Then when you have a low moment or you want to give up, just go through those reasons in your mind, and it will really help.

Number **one**, running helps me lose weight. Number **two**, running helps me to get healthy. Number **three**, running relieves my stress. Number **four**, running gives me a chance to think about the day ahead. **Five**, running makes me revitalized and awake well before I'm in the office. **Six**, running will help me to live longer. **Seven**, running means I get to explore my local area and neighborhood. **Eight**, running means I can go back to refereeing soccer if I want. **Nine**, running means I will lose weight and, therefore, have a greater selection of nice suits to choose from. Number **ten**, running should lead to me losing weight and being attractive to the opposite sex. Come on. I had to have one laddish one in there.

Running so I could lose weight and buy more clothes (number nine) was inspirational, because I was fed up going to the fat-guy store. Or I'd walk past a designer store, and I would go in there and really admire these wonderful suits, knowing I wouldn't even ask if they had it in my size because they never did. Have you noticed that? They don't carry your size. So then you have to go to specialty stores. I used that as a mechanism for getting me juicing and running and getting healthy.

Another thing I did was I put some money away every month, because what I wanted to do when I hit my goal weight was to hire a personal shopper who would interview me, find out my likes, my dislikes, go out, and pick out a load of clothes. Then I would meet her, and we'd go try them all on. It was very indulgent, but that was my goal. And I did it.

I put the money away every month. It wasn't a financial hardship because obviously it took me a while to get to the 70-pound loss. I went out with Rachel, a personal shopper, and bought a new wardrobe. It felt amazing that I could wear these very nice suits and trousers, and I could wear the attractive shirts that previously I couldn't because they didn't make them for fat guys.

So this visualization is a vital part of the process. As I was out there running in negative 30-degree weather, I would just go over these reasons in my head, and it would keep me going. Now, I'm 80 pounds lighter as a result of having these positive thoughts in my mind. So it's very important. For you, it could be swimming. It could be walking. It could just be the juicing, whatever works for you.

I visualized myself finishing the Stockholm half-marathon. And, interestingly enough, it took me three years to do that because I moved around the world. But I went back to Sweden and I ran that half-marathon. I really wish you could have met me in 2010. You've seen the photographs. I was incredibly overweight. I certainly couldn't run. It was amazing to return to Stockholm and run and complete that in a really good time—I broke two hours. That was my goal, and I did it. In Sweden I was able to look certain people in the eye, who told me that juicing was a fad, and I would never lose the weight or I'd never be able to run 5K, let alone a half-marathon.

Sometimes you can use these almost confrontational points to help you get through your journey. So that's Train Your Brain. Let's move to the last two.

Sixth Key—Shift

Change your routine. On my first juice fast, I started running. I use that word "running" lightly. I did the Couch Potato to 5K, a great program and I highly recommend it if you want to start running. It's one of these programs where you walk two minutes, run one minute. Over eight weeks, it gets you to be able to run for 30 minutes nonstop—it's a wonderful program.

Angie, my delightful co-host on Juicing Radio, started swimming. If you sit at home like a hermit during your reboot, it can be difficult, because your mind starts thinking about food and eating and social stuff. It's good to break up your routine a little bit. What you'll find is that because you're not cooking, you'll have a lot more time in the evening. That's when your mind can play tricks on you. So Angie went swimming. I went running. Maybe there's some kind of meet-up group you want to attend or do some charity work. Whatever it is, try to break up your routine, if possible, and it will be a big help.

Seventh Key—Don't Be Afraid to Be Different

You can be an innovator here. What I mean is if the juice recipes or the plan you're following are not doing it for you, then feel free to mix things up. As long as you try to stick to the 80 percent veggies, 20 percent fruit, you'll be all right. What's fascinating is with almost 60 interviews of success stories on Juicing Radio, nearly every single one of those people free-styled to begin their juicing. By free-styled, I mean they followed the program for a couple of days and then experimented some.

Our friend Shawna in San Francisco, for instance, didn't like the pineapple in the Jason Vale recipe. Cool. Substitute it with more kale or some pear. Mix it up a little bit. Try something else that tastes better on your palate or gives you more energy, makes you feel vibrant. You don't have to stick to the regimen.

I remember the first couple of days I did stick to a recipe, because I was a little bit scared that if I put in melon I might get sick. Because let's be honest. It's a whole new experience for many of us, but you can freestyle. Generally those are the people who are the most successful.

So I want to end with a quote. This is all very serious, right? Our health is serious. When you undertake a juice fast, it is serious business, because you've got a really important goal that could change your life for good, but remember the following words.

> **Laugh and have fun.**
> **Reach for the mountaintop,**
> **but enjoy the climb.**

I have to tell you I enjoyed my climb. I had low points. I'm not going to lie. There were struggles, but I'm really enjoying being on top of the mountaintop and being 80 pounds lighter.

I love the fact I can go out now and run. I've just signed up to play soccer again for a team in New York City. I don't think my soccer skills have improved, but at least I know I'll be able to run around the field and be able to keep up with everyone. The mountaintop, it's a great view.

So you keep on with your climb! The very fact you're reading these keys for successful juicing—if you put these into practice, you are soon going to be on the mountaintop. I want you to email me when you're on top of that mountain and tell me what the view is like. Or if you're struggling on your climb, get in touch with me. Shane@juicingradio.com. I'd love to hear from you, would love to help you, because this is what we do at Juicing Radio, because that view from the mountaintop is spectacular. Good luck.

Get your free copy of
How to Get Started with Juicing
**and receive free email juice coaching
(but not spam—that's not healthy).**

Sign up at www.juicinghabits.com.

JUICING RADIO

Shane and Angie invite you to listen to a juicing success story every week on Juicing Radio.

Sign up for updates and never miss an episode at JuicingRadio.com.

Thank Goodness for Juicing Radio!

by LA Juice Girl

I just started juicing after listening to Shane and Angie on Juicing Radio a couple weeks ago, and I have already completed a juice fast and I am now juicing daily. The podcast is informative, entertaining, and very motivating, especially for juicing newbies like me! I would highly recommend Juicing Radio as they are definitely one of the top resources for juicers worldwide.

Joe Cross Talks about his Health Journey and How He's Not Perfect

Introduction to the Interview

Are you interested in juicing, but never tried? Are you in the middle of a juice fast or just about to transition to a balanced diet? Whatever your stage, Juicing Radio, brings you the industry experts, success stories, latest news and recipes; gives useful tips and resources; and inspires and empowers you to change your life for good. Welcome your first host, an ordinary guy who managed to lose 80 pounds while running on juice, juice fanatic Shane Whaley. And your second host is Angie von Buelow, who lost 86 pounds and has been promoting the benefits of juicing!

Shane: Hi and welcome to Juicing Radio. Today's guest needs little introduction. Chances are you're drinking a green juice because of him. Chances are you went out and bought a juicer because of him. Chances are your local juice bar opened because of him, and chances are you listened to Juicing Radio because of him. Welcome, Joe Cross.

Joe: Thanks, Shane. Thanks, Angie. It's great to be here—love being here—what you guys are doing is great and I love listening. Now I'm on the show and I'm really excited.

Shane: Well, we're excited to have you here, and we can all talk juicing. Each of us lost more than 80 pounds. We've all been on great journeys, but what we decided to do was to go to our listeners, we have 4,000 a week now, and ask them to submit questions. Last night at Barnes and Noble in New York City, you gave a great talk.

Joe: Thank you.

Shane: Lots of people wanted to ask you questions, so we wanted to give our audience the opportunity to do that. One of the questions I wanted to ask you is this. When you filmed *Fat, Sick and Nearly Dead* and when you launched the movie, did you have any idea how big it was going to be?

Joe: I had no idea at all, Shane. When I made the movie I thought maybe a few thousand, maybe 10,000 people might buy the DVD or they might watch the movie, stay at a retreat on top of a mountain where people are sipping ginger tea. I thought it would be a very niche subject—this big, fat Australian guy goes and drinks juice for 60 days. Little did I know what journey I would be on. Little did I know the impact that this movie would have on regular people. So the movie became something that got ahead of me, and I had to sort of build a business and a community around it, because of the outreach, the continual question about "What's in the juice? What's this?"

I mean, I'll give you an example. When I was trying to sell the movie I went out to Hollywood and I played the movie to several studios. After every screening a round of applause, standing ovation, and I'm thinking, "This is good. I'm going to sell it." The executive would come up and say, "Listen, that was fantastic. What sort of juicer was that, and what's the recipe?"

And I'd tell him that, and then I would say, "So I guess you want to buy the movie?"

He goes, "Oh, no, no. You're not Hugh Jackman or Russell Crowe. We don't know how to sell the movie, but we want the juicer and we want the recipe. We've all got to lose a few pounds. We've all got to get healthy."

So in the end I had to really make my own way. I had to find a way to get the movie out, and I got lucky through the power of social media—through the power of YouTube and through the power of Netflix streaming. I think what the movie did was fill a void that was out there in terms of information, inspiration, and entertainment. When you have those three things together packaged up in a non-preachy way, where it's just about getting out there and doing it and not telling people what to do, I think that even I am surprised. I'm surprised by the amount of success it has had, but when you put all that together, you can see why.

Shane: Absolutely. It's a very inspiring movie.

Joe: Thank you, mate.

Angie: Here's a question that I have. What do you eat these days, Joe? Everyone wants to know.

Shane: Because you're not juicing anymore, right? You made the movie how many years ago?

Joe: The movie was made about six years ago. That's when I wrapped it. I get asked that question a lot, "What do I eat today?" I eat a lot more plant food than I used to eat. I am really big on making sure that every meal I have, there are plants present—fruits, vegetables, nuts, beans, and seeds. Some days I'm really, really good at getting about 40 percent of the total energy I consume that day from plants. But about 40 to 50 days out of the whole year, I take a big pitcher. I will only juice or eat plant food. So I guess the way that I am approaching it is that I've learned a lot and I'm on a journey, and I am by no means perfect. There are certain things I don't eat at all. I don't drink a lot of sodas and I don't eat certain processed foods.

I won't go to a chain restaurant and eat food. But I will have a healthy hamburger at someone's house, if it's made in the backyard on the barbecue. For many years after I made the movie I didn't eat any meat, but then recently I started eating some. I have a lot of fish. If I'm going to eat an animal, that's what I eat the most. I don't drink coffee. I don't drink a lot of soda, but every now and then on special occasions I will have a ginger ale. I drink a lot of water. I drink a lot of fresh juice. I don't drink a lot of tea, but sometimes in cold weather I will have herbal teas.

I don't smoke cigarettes anymore, and I really try to limit the foods that are white. Pasta is a very, very rare thing for me to have. Gluten-free bread is what I'm eating lately, and that's sort of working. But in all of this I'm not perfect, and there are days where I'm not where I should be, but I accept that. I don't beat myself up. I just think, "You know what? Tomorrow I'm going to be better. I'm going to be like a hunter-gatherer. I'm going to get out there and I'm going to try to find my plants."

I find that if I start my day with lots of plants—be it a juice, be it a smoothie, be it a fruit salad—and then move into salads for lunch, that by the time dinner has come along, if I've lived on plants all day, I feel good. Mentally I'm very strong, and so on the back of that I can then go out that evening and not get too crazy; but I might have some fish, I might have some rice (if I'm doing sushi), or I might have some chicken.

Angie: I think it's so important to start your day with the juice. I find that I make healthier choices throughout the day.

Joe: I think if you put the juice in early, what you're effectively doing is putting the nutrients from the plant into your body and your cells are being fed. If you can get your cells fed early in day, they're not going to be loud and boisterous and sort of complaining, and slamming their hands on the table saying, "Feed me!" You're going to be less hungry.

I think today is a good example. I've had three juices already and I had a tomato with avocado salad and a little bit of grilled chicken. I'm actually quite satisfied.

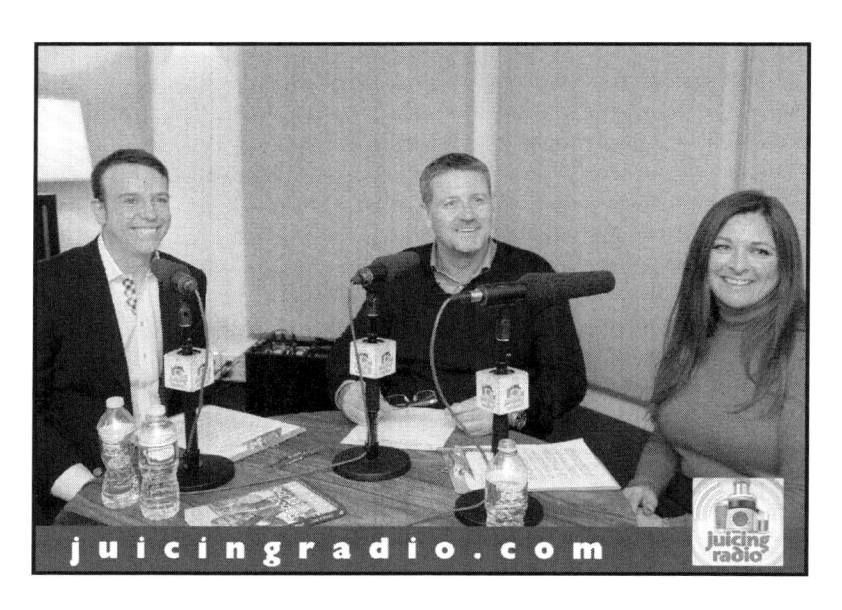

Shane: You said something in your talk last night that really struck a chord with me. You were talking about being on the road and you go into a place to eat. You see on one side the burgers. Another side you see the pizza and the salad in the middle, and you automatically want the salad. You've conditioned yourself to look at the salad and go for it. I often find, even though I've gone through a similar journey, that I'm still kind of drawn to that. "Oh, that cheeseburger looks pretty good," but really, I know I should have the tomato and mozzarella. I thought that was really important how you have conditioned yourself to go for the salad side of the menu rather than the other food.

Joe: I think the point I was making was that we all have choices in life. When you look at any menu and see what's offered, our eyes will always find the things that are appealing and the most attractive to us. Say that there is a choice between a cheeseburger and a salad. In the old days, the conversation inside my head went something like this: "I know the salad is better for me, but I want the cheeseburger. Should I have the salad? But I really want the cheeseburger."

I would have this back and forth dilemma, maybe half a dozen times in the space of 20 seconds. Then I say, "You know what? I'll be good tomorrow. I'm having the cheeseburger," and I would order the cheeseburger. That's the old days.

The new days are like this: I see the cheeseburger and I see the salad. I think, "How long has it been since I had a cheeseburger? I had one last week. Well, how have I been lately? Is this the place I really want to have that cheeseburger? Is this a place that's going to be so great that I'm really missing out on not having that cheeseburger? Because, actually, I'm pretty excited about the salad."

So it's not such a difficult decision. I say, "You know what? I'll take the salad." Quite often I'll ask the people in the restaurant, "Please tell me, how good are the salads here? What's the best salad that you're serving? What's the most popular salad? If you had to eat a salad, what would you eat?" Because they're working there. They know. If they reply, "Listen, the salads here are pretty ordinary. Limp this and that. It's not good."

Then that might be a place that I say, "Well, tell me about the cheeseburger." So I'll really investigate and get some buy in from the supplier, even the person working the floor or the restaurant owner, or whatever. Whereas in the old days I never used to ask what was good. I never used to ask, "What would you eat?" I used to just come in and my eyes would level down. I would see the food that is white, brown, or black, that had high processed flour, sugar, salt, and I would just instantly be attracted to that.

Shane: You've got 4,000 people nodding their heads at that right now, I'm sure.

Joe: Only 4,000? Add a zero to that.

Shane: Yeah, absolutely.

Angie: Well, let's get to some of our questions from our listeners. First we have a question on behalf of a Facebook group, Juicing for Dummies. This is from Christy Whitley. "I want to know where Joe first heard about juicing. Who inspired him?"

Joe: When you say "first heard about juicing," obviously juicing is something that, in Australia, there were lots of juice bars, so there was lots of juicing going on. But I think what Christy is asking or referring to is probably, "Where did you come up with this idea of juice fasting? Where did that idea come from?" And to be quite honest, I actually don't know where I first heard of the words "juice fasting." I know that I remember reading a book that was a 1971 edition by an Italian doctor. It had about 500 pages, but there were 3 pages on juice fasting.

Before that what I did was looked at this idea of merging the two, which was, I'm fat and I'm sick. Why am I fat? Because I'm holding on to all this energy to use up for lean times. So the solution there is to just drink water. So I've got that covered. Then I looked at the sick. I'm sick. Why am I sick? Because I've turned my back on Mother Nature. I just need to eat lots of plants, lots of food that she makes, fruits, vegetables, nuts, beans, and seeds. So now I have this problem because I'm supposed to, on the one hand, lose the weight, not eat, but, on the other hand, to get well from being sick was to eat all these plants. So I kind of compromised. I said, "What if I extract the water from the plants? What if I could somehow get the water out of the cucumber, get the water out of the celery, get the water out of the apples, the oranges, the pears, and other fruits and vegetables? What if I could take all that water and only drink the water from plants?

That, in essence, is what juicing is. It's drinking water filtered through plants. So then I had this idea about a two-year regimen where I only eat plants to find out if I could cure myself from my autoimmune disease, which everybody was effectively saying that I was going to have for the rest of my life. People would tell me, "This is idiopathic, Joe. We don't know what caused it. We don't know how to heal you, but you've got to take these pills, and that's just it, mate. Suck it up. We'll have to monitor you, and da, da, da, da."

Well, that was outsourcing my help. So when I took back control and brought the health in-house, so to speak, at that point I needed the plan. The plan was that if I can drink water filtered through juice for 60 days to kick off my two-year journey, then that might be a great way to supercharge my body, give my body the nutrients it needs with all the information that's contained in these micronutrients. Then I've got to eat lots of other food later and be excited about it, and hopefully my taste buds would be rebooted, which is exactly what happened.

Shane: Fantastic. Jocelyn Aria asks a really fascinating question, Joe, because your message is about promoting the eating and drinking of more fruits and veggies to as many people as you can. She asks if *Fat, Sick and Nearly Dead* will be made available in other languages. I think she is in Quebec. I lived in Sweden, and the Swedes are pretty good at English, but I know there are a lot of non-English speaking people, who prefer to watch movies in their own language. So in terms of really further promoting your message, have you considered subtitles in other languages?

Joe: Yes, in fact, we've actually got the film subtitled into 15 different languages right now. So that's really exciting. Now, the issue is getting it distributed. I had a meeting with a team of guys who told me that Netflix is moving into Germany and France, so with the power of these corporations that are getting out there with streaming content, that's going to be great new markets.

How do you get the message out? How do you get the word out? Doing the subtitles is easy. It's not very expensive. You get it done, you get it wrapped, so we've got it in 15 languages, and I know we've got a French version. So, Jocelyn we did have the movie on YouTube in Canada with subtitles not so long ago, and it might still be on, if you want to check. And there are DVDs for sale that have the subtitles.

Angie: We have another question. It's from Isabella Russel, and she's from the United Kingdom. "How do you introduce juicing to someone who needs it, but is very skeptical about it?"

Joe: That's a really good question, and I don't really have an answer, because every one of us is different. I think by example. I think that Isabella has to do it herself. She has to show the person she cares about, what the impact of drinking fresh fruit and vegetable juice can have on her, and show that person. I think if there's a way of somehow saying, "Hey, let's do something together. Let's get a group of four or five of us. We'd love you to join and be a part of it, but not in a way that we're trying to look after you. I'm asking you to join to help me."

I think the best way to learn is to teach, and when you do that and encourage someone, not with all the focus on them, then they're part of something and they have an opportunity to inspire others—I think that can also help. But it's a good question I get asked from many people.

"You know, Joe, my son, my dad, my mother, my daughter, my sister, my brother, all need your help. We would love you to put them in the next movie." I can understand how people's hopes are dashed and they're trying to look after the people they love. I get it. I wish I could clone myself and go to all these places and do that. I would love nothing more. It's just not all about me. It's about those people inside having this motivation to go from what we call the "knowing" to the "doing," and that step, it's very easy to say, but it's not as easy to put into practice. But it's much easier when they see people who are doing it, when they're part of a group that's doing it, and they're made to feel that they're not on their own.

Shane: And I think, if I can add to that point, something that we've talked about a lot is not preaching to people. I've made this mistake in the past: where I've dropped the 80 pounds, I'm feeling good, I'm running half marathons, and I'm living in the bubble, right? I'm in the juicing bubble, and I'm almost lecturing. I've lost friends over this, right?

They're like, "Shut up, Shane. I've had enough of this juicing stuff." So it's really important that people see our own transformations and come to us. That's something you were able to do, Joe. My parents even saw my transformation. They still eat meat and potatoes and everything else, and all of a sudden I was on channel five in the United Kingdom. I get an email from my mother, which said, "Oh, me and your dad are doing a three-day juice fast."

So you were able to go where I couldn't as their own son, right?

Joe: We had the luxury of looking at it 500 times to make sure that the tone was right and all those things. Yes, I understand the people preachers, I think there's a group of people who love listening to preachers once a week on a Sunday, and I respect that, and that's somewhere where it works. But I think in everyday life among our friends and family, being told what to do doesn't work. And I think that it's all about getting out there, leading by example, and sharing when people ask. When somebody asks, it's not to ram it down their throat. It's like saying, "Hey, listen. I'm glad you're interested. If you want any help, I'll help. If you want to do something, it's great."

Women are very good at this. Women are natural nurturers. Men are a little bit more about, "You've got to do this, mate, this is what you've got to do! You've got to do this!" We get excited, and I can understand that. And by the way, when you've lost a lot of weight, or when you've regained your health, because you feel so fabulous and you feel alive and you feel young and you feel focused, sometimes that enthusiasm can get a little bit mixed up for preaching, when it's really not. You're just super excited to share the love and the knowledge. I even get accused of that.

Shane: Great. So our next question is asked by Paula in North Carolina. She says, "I'm new to juicing. If we don't like a lot of veggies, is it okay to juice a lot of fruit with a little veggies? Thanks for everything you've done."

Joe: So, Paula, here's what I would say. I would say that each of us is different. There are 320 million people in America. There's 22 or 23 million where I come from. I think the United Kingdom has about 60 million. We're all different. We've all got different ways to approach our food. You sound like you've got a bit of a sweet tooth, which is understandable. You're not in the minority. You're in the majority. So start out that way. Start out putting more fruit in. But make this commitment to yourself that over time, maybe over a month it will take, that you're 80 percent fruit and 20 percent veggies. Maybe after one week it will get down to 60/40. Maybe the next week it's at 50/50, and maybe the next week you will be able to finally kick the veggies up a little bit more.

And maybe it plateaus there for a month. Maybe you can't make anymore changes, or you try to do something else and it doesn't work. So I would really be your own taste tester and be your own nutritional gatekeeper, in that it's very important that we can train our bodies to have less sugar. The taste will come.

Just think about this, Paula. If you were on a desert island for five weeks and all you had was water, and I turned up with a cucumber juice and nothing else in it, that would be the best drink you've ever had in your life. Because for five weeks on water, to finally taste something else? Oh, that cucumber juice would be unbelievable. So it's about where you come from. It's very difficult to drink something, such as a Mountain Dew or a Sprite or some kind of cola, if you then go and have a juice. You're just not going to get the same heightened senses. That bliss point is just not going to be there. So it's okay to start out, but you don't want to stay there. If you're doing that constantly, you'll disrupt your pancreas and put yourself at risk of becoming a diabetic, and we don't want that.

Angie: Our next question is from Debbie Shields. "I watched Joe's movie, *Fat, Sick and Nearly Dead.* Currently I'm doing a 60-day reboot and would like to know if Joe exercised every day when he did his reboot. If he did, what did he do and for how long?"

Joe: Debbie, when you're making a movie it's a lot of work, and you're standing around waiting for all the sounds dudes, the camera dudes, and the producers to get the things right, so you do a lot of standing, you do a lot of walking, and they were long days. I was up before the sunrise and not to bed until late after sunset. So the answer is I didn't really do any specific routine program every day. There were days when I did lots of hikes. I did some exercise, such as swimming and some weights, but generally there wasn't a set routine.

After the 60 days of juicing and doing my journey on the 90 days of eating plants, I was then doing a lot of exercise. I had an hour a day and a trainer, and I was visiting a gym on a regular basis about six days a week. I was really interested and excited. I find with my workouts that when I'm on, I'm on; and when I'm off, I'm really off.

So that's what I did during the 60 days of juicing. It's not really advisable to lift weights while you're juicing unless you're substituting with some kind of plant protein, because you're not really putting enough protein into your body. The idea of a juice fast or a reboot or a period of time of just drinking juice is not a sustainable way to live the rest of your life. It's a period of time to say, "You know what? I'm going to take a trip back in time. I'm going to go back to a time when there wasn't any food around. I'm going to create a nutritional famine. I'm going to just purely live on the water that is filtered through plants, and I'm going to trick my body. Yes, trick it into thinking it's only drinking water. But I'm actually putting in these tens of thousands of nutrients and harnessed, captured sun. I'm going to drink it, and I'm going to give my body the nourishment, the information, the science that it needs to stay healthy and pure, and it's only going to be a short period of time."

I think that I talked about this last night that the jury is out, but will come back with a good verdict on the fact that fasting is a part of human nature. Look at all the big religions. You've got Christianity, Muslim, Hindu, and Buddhism. They all have fasting in them, and a lot of other religions also have it. But they're the big four with the populations around the world. So fasting is part of our history. It's part of human nature. Look at animals—when they don't eat, it indicates that they're a bit sick. For babies, not eating is a way that they communicate to parents that they're not well.

It's a very, very normal and natural thing to do. I don't believe that we have the ability to gain all of this energy and walk around with so much energy in our bodies if there wasn't a purpose for saving it up for lean times.

Shane: This is from Jamie Robinson, who is with the Sydney, Australia, vegan club. Jamie says, "Australia, much like the United Kingdom, has alcohol engrained in its culture. Every event, even finishing work for the day, warrants a cold one. What tips do you have to overcome social pressures and expectations?"

Joe: Well, I don't drink alcohol anymore. I haven't had a drink since the night before I filmed the movie when I had a few beers. It was sort of saying goodbye to food for the next 60 days I've had no wine, no alcohol, no spirits, no nothing in the past six-and-a-half years. I love the idea of having this mental clarity of just not ever being a little bit tipsy or in any way impaired by alcohol. I love it. I don't miss alcohol one bit. I don't ever think, "I would love a drink."

I mean, there have been times during the years when I've been sitting on friends' boats and there have been beautiful sunsets. I've thought, "That would be nice to have that taste," but I can count the times on one hand. And that's pretty good in six-and-a-half years.

Now, I don't *not* drink because I think drinking is bad for you. That's not the reason why I don't drink. I don't drink because I just like having the clarity. In the old days when I would have two or three drinks, sometimes I couldn't stop. It wasn't like I was an alcoholic, but I just enjoyed it so much. I'm a big, loud, gregarious, fun guy and that included topping off my glass, and before I knew it I'd had seven or eight—then it's going to turn into twenty.

That sets up the next day to not feel good, to be a bit down on myself, and then the food choices I'm going to make the next day are going to trigger a whole series of events that I'm not going to be happy with or proud of that could send me into a spiral for a week or two. So that's why I've sort of decided not to drink alcohol any more.

That doesn't mean that you won't run into me somewhere down at Bondi Beach, Jamie, and I'm having a beer next year. I'm not saying that I'm never going to drink again. I'm saying so far, as of today, I haven't felt like a drink.

So how do you deal with the social pressure? Well, I know what Australia is like, and it is quite incredible just how much people drink there. I was in England last week, and they're big drinkers there. So I heard something interesting that someone told me. They said, "You know what? If you can go two days a week, one week a month and one month a year without a drink, that's a nice, balanced way to live your life."

So think about that—two days a week, one week a month, one month a year. So what I would say to Jamie with respect to alcohol is, "Moderation is perfect." I think that if friends are upset or angry, you're sort of turning a mirror on them and they're seeing themselves, and they think that you're better than them and they start to have a go at you. I get it. I think that you've got to think about the perspective of how important your health is to you, and ask them to respect that.

If at the end of the day they don't, and they're giving you too much grief, well, mate, you're probably not going to want to hang out with these people. They're not going to be the sort of friends that you're going to associate with going forward. If it's a personal thing that you feel you want to have a drink to participate because you can't have fun, then maybe what you do is just start with one glass of champagne and try to make it last the whole night. That's how I would approach it.

Shane: In your book, Joe, you mention that you don't drink Coca-Cola anymore either. My question is this. Let's say Sydney Swans are playing and we all go down to the pub to watch. What do you drink? You're not drinking Coke, and you're not drinking booze.

Joe: If we've gone to see a game in the pub, and I say, "I've eaten plants in the morning, I've had my juices, and I've gone for a walk or run on the beach," then I might have a lime and soda or I might have a ginger ale. A lime and soda for me is club soda with fresh lime juice. I don't like the lime cordial. I like the lime juice from fresh limes. You take a whole lime, you squeeze it, you get about half an inch of juice in the bottom of a glass and then lots of ice and club soda. Mix it up. It's a great drink.

But if that's not available then I go to the ginger ale. Now, I know the ginger ale has high fructose corn syrup in it. I know that. I think it has a bit of caffeine in it too, so it's a very rare thing that I will have a ginger ale.

Shane: It's something I've often wondered. I'm a huge football fan. When I started juicing I gave up booze for 14 months—coming from Britain, that was a big deal.

Joe: Oh, a big deal.

Shane: But it was the juicing. I didn't wake up and say, "I don't want a drink." It was the juicing that made me make those healthier choices. But now when I go to the bar I don't want to drink Coca-Cola. My weakness is actually root beer. I did smile when I was reading your book. I disciplined myself to have only one on a Saturday night, and if I remember, your temptation, especially when you're in London, is chocolate ice cream.

Joe: Yeah, I love chocolate ice cream. I guess the two things that I used to love the most were Coca-Cola and chocolate ice cream, and when you put chocolate ice cream in Coca-Cola . . .

Angie: Sweet. Coke floats. That's where it's at.

Joe: Is that what it's called?

Angie: Coke float. Yeah.

Joe: But going back to Coca-Cola for a second, I don't think that Coca-Cola is bad for you. I don't look at it as the enemy. I know that for me, if I drink Coca-Cola, I'm worried that I would want to have more than just one. It's the sort of thing for me that has so many memories, so much connection, so much history, because I used to drink a lot of it.

I was 14 when my grandfather died, and he was an alcoholic. For the last 20 years of his life, he had never had a drink. We used to talk about it. I used to speak to my grandfather Tuesday night and Friday night for three or four years from the age of 10 to 14, and we would talk about it.

He would say, "You know, Joe, you want to watch your drinking. It didn't do me any good."

I said, "Yeah, yeah. Sure, Grandpa. Let's get on to talk about something else." I mean, I was 12. What are you going to tell me about alcohol for? I'm 12. But when he passed away and I was at his funeral, I made a pledge that I wouldn't drink alcohol until I was 18 in his honor and his name.

I left school when I was 17. All through high school I never drank. Even one year out, when I was working (I didn't go to university or college), I was six months into my work year when I had my first beer. I never had any alcohol, and because I drank soda so much I was drinking lots of Coke. So we would go to restaurants as big groups, as you do when you're teenagers, with about 20 people at a time. I would have maybe seven or eight cans of Coke at dinner.

Angie: That's a lot of Coke.

Joe: Oh, yeah. I was just like everyone else. I was hyped up and ready to go because I've got the sugar and the caffeine, and I could drive home, which was great.

Angie: You're popular.

Joe: Then when it came to dividing the bill up among 20 people, because everyone is half sloshed, I divided by 19. So it was perfect.

Angie: You were a smart guy at an early age.

Joe: I was a smart guy. I didn't pay for a meal for two years. So the reality is that Coca-Cola has this history for me of not just having a Coke—it's having lots of Coke. So maybe one day, if I get confident and strong enough, I could go back to having one Coke after a game of golf or doing something. But for the moment I've decided to just keep it at bay. I'm doing okay.

Shane: A lot of the questions we're asking you today you've answered in your book. Can you tell us what prompted you to write this book? It's called *The Reboot with Joe Juice Diet: Lose Weight, Get Healthy, and Feel Amazing*.

Joe: Well, it's basically driven by the tens of thousands, if not hundreds of thousands, of people who are really interested in having the whole A to Z—what to do, how to do it, and to hear it from my words and my mouth to their ears. So I probably should have written this book at the time the movie came out, but I had no idea, as I said earlier, about the success of the movie. I had no idea it was going to end up that way. So I think that I've been chasing the community. I've been behind and the community has gotten out ahead of me.

They've all been asking for information. They've all wanted stuff, and I've just been sort of trying my best. So I thought that I needed infrastructure. I need a team. I need a bunch of people and I need to get more money, and we had the economic crisis going on and things were tough. So it took a while to get all this in place. It's only really now, and I said this to the team the other day, I really think it's only in the last three to six months that we finally not only caught up, but we actually got out in front.

When you have a community with millions of people who are interested in following and listening and knowing what you do, it's important not to get too far out in front. You don't want to be ten steps ahead, or you'll leave them behind. You just want to be a step ahead. I feel like I've been two or three steps behind, and so now we're a step ahead, and that's a comfortable place. On the back of that, this film has spawned this book for all the new people.

Right now, somewhere in the world, someone is watching *Fat, Sick and Nearly Dead* for the first time. So the lucky thing for them (as opposed to Angie and Shane, when you saw the movie there wasn't a handbook), now there is a book with the knowledge that I know about my journey about juicing—what to do on a reboot, what to do after a reboot, and lots of success stories that you know only too well.

Shane: Angie's one of those success stories.

Joe: She is indeed. Fantastic story. It just goes to show that from my point of view, to sit on the side that I sit on, to know that through my illness (I was walking around for eight years, tripping over my bottom lip, saying, "Why me? Why me?") I was able to somehow, don't know how, but I was able to manifest that real negative thing in my life into such a positive. It's the best thing that has ever happened to me. I mean, I haven't had kids yet, and I'm pretty confident that when I have kids that will be the best thing. But for now the best thing that is happening in my life is to see the change and the effect that my story (and the story that's illustrated by Phil Staples and others in the movie, in the community, and in this book) can pay it forward and continue to affect other people's health and happiness, and that's a really cool thing.

Angie: You have a second movie coming out, right? Can you share a bit about that?

Joe: The new movie is *Fat, Sick and Nearly Dead 2.* There you go. That's a really original name, but a lot of these people know the first movie, and I want to capitalize on the brand. *Fat, Sick and Nearly Dead 2* picks up the story six years later.

I originally said I wouldn't make another movie, but I chose to just because of the amount of interest. At the time, I didn't want to after what I had been through, and, remember, the movie hadn't been out when I said those words. I didn't know it was going to be as big as it was, and I didn't know there would be a reason to make another one. I waited six years because I haven't really had a story to tell. But I think now there's more of an interesting story as to what's going on here. Why is it happening? Why is it working for some people and not for others? How important is community?

Let's say that you were one of the people in the movie who I went up and spoke to. What was it like for them three years ago, two years ago, when the movie broke and all their friends started ringing them up and saying, "We saw you in this movie!" What happens to them when they see themselves in the context of all of these people who are sort of going along with their lives, not really looking at their priories?

I mean, I was focusing on everything else but my health. So it has been great to reconnect with some of those people I met and see what impact the movie has had on them, on others, and this story now is continuing. We're already working on movie number three and hopefully a fourth. I think that the story of plants—and how we have turned our backs on them, and how powerful they can be for us in going forward—has been around a long time. But I still believe that it can be told many ways, many times, through the eyes of lots of interesting, fun, and intelligent people.

Shane: I always urge people to buy the actual DVD. Because of the bonus special features!

Joe: There are 90 minutes of special features and the director's commentary, which I need to listen to again. We had a lot of fun making that.

Shane: I can imagine.

Angie: The director's commentary is one of my favorite parts of the DVD.

Joe: Kurt Engfehr, the director, and I are talking and chatting about the whole thing.

Angie: The story of how you actually made the movie, the journey of that, is fascinating.

Shane: I always find it very useful. When I was on a reboot, I wanted as much good information as I could get about juicing and reboot. So I would watch the movie first. Then the next night, I would watch the 90 minutes of bonus features, especially that lady in the Laundromat. She will always stick with me.

Joe: For those who haven't seen this part, let me explain. I walked into a Laundromat. There was a lovely lady there with her son. She was doing her laundry and I had to do mine. She was on the larger side of life. She had a lot of energy that her body was hanging onto, waiting for the next famine.

I had a chat with her. She told me that she was on half a dozen, maybe even more, medications, and when I talked to her about her size, I said, "Do you think that there's anything wrong with being the way you are?"

She said, "No, no, no. It has been in the family. God made me this way. God made me this way."

And it's hard to argue with that, you know? Someone who is very, very religious, someone who has strong faith and believes that the reason why she was large was because God made her that way. So I respected that. Then when we started talking about her health and she talked about these pills, I actually asked her the question, "Do you think God made you so that you would take the seven or eight medications a day?"

She paused. She actually thought about it. She said, "No, probably not."

That was a real interesting opener for her that she actually now connected her size and the way that she was to her health, which is kind of obvious for lots of people. But there are lots of people who don't actually get that connection. So that's okay.

Anyway, she was a lovely lady and her son was a lot of fun. He was cool and it was nice to meet them. But that was a scene that didn't make it into the movie. It was originally, but then it ended up on the cutting-room floor, because we had so much other incredible content to share.

The special features are fun with 90 minutes and the director's commentary all on the DVD.

Shane: So buy a copy of the DVD. It really helps, especially when you're on a reboot. It's extra content for you.

Joe, let's go back to your book. First, I think you've been refreshingly honest in your book. There are a lot of diet books, should we say, or health-and-wellness books in which I don't think the author is as honest as you have been. Even last night in your talk you were saying, "Look, I'm not perfect." You're trying your best and you're not perfect.

Joe: No. I can't stand perfect people.

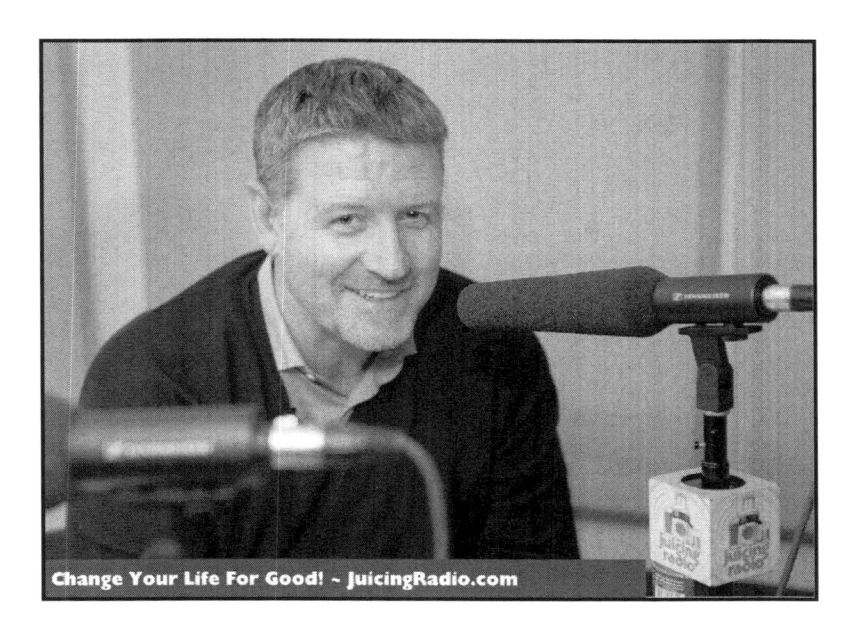

Shane: Absolutely, and I think that is why you have been so successful. People resonate with you, Joe. You're very down to earth, and that comes across in the movie, the way you speak to people and the way you're carrying the message.

Now, there were lots of important concepts in the book, but one particular thing really struck me. Would you talk us through what it was like for you? You've done the 60 days, you've been up in the hot air balloon, you fly home to Sydney, you see your parents for the first time, right? From day 1 to day 60, you hadn't seen them in that time. What was that like? Can you talk us through what happened?

Joe: I was teased all around. Mom and Dad were really happy. It was great to look good, and they were amazed. My mum said I looked 10, 15, 20 years younger, something like that. But I was on medication, even though the dose was lower, I was still on the pills. So I told them, "This is great, but I've now got to keep this going. I've got to get off these pills, and I don't know how long that's going to take. I've just got to keep persevering with just the plants and the juice." I think that they were really excited for me and happy to see me look healthy and happy and feel full of energy.

However, I said, "You should do this."

"Oh, no, we're not doing that. We're not doing that. We're not going anywhere near that. We're not doing the juicing."

And it wasn't until later, when they saw themselves in the film, after the movie came out, that they said, "We're definitely going to do it."

So they did their first reboot after the movie. So even with me (relating back to what you said earlier, Shane), my parents had to wait until the movie came out to begin juicing.

Shane: Incredible.

Joe: I think that they were happier, to be honest, 90 days later when I told them that I was off all medication. I think that's when they were more excited. I've got to be honest—I was more excited about being medication free. I remember the day that I didn't take the pills. It was 90 days later. I had decreased the medication with a doctor's supervision to go to zero.

I lasted the day and it was fine. I lasted another day, and I didn't get excited. I didn't rush out and do the filming. I waited. I wanted to wait a whole week, because I was really worried that a flare-up would occur, or some condition would happen. So I waited. Then after a week, I asked my assistant at the time (Alex Hoarder, a great girl in Sydney who was working for me) to film me. She had never operated a camera before in her life, but I said, "Alex, I'm going to show you what to do. You're going to climb out into the surf with me at Bondi Beach, and part of your job description is to film Joe taking a dive under a wave."

Alex was great. She kept the camera dry. She got drenched, but that was all right. We did the shot, and I walked along the beach barefoot for the first time, not having to wear any footwear. I could actually walk barefoot on the beach.

Before, that uneven pressure on my feet through the sand and having all that pressure of my body going through to one point would cause my feet to swell. So that's what I was super excited about, and it was only then that I really felt we had something in the movie that would be really, really exciting.

Angie: I think people aren't aware of how debilitating the diseases that you were suffering from were, and how it really impacted every aspect of your life.

Joe: Yeah, it was terrible. I often say to people, "I've got really soft hands," because for eight years I couldn't use them. I wasn't able to do any physical labor. I'm a big guy. I would go to someone's house, and they would ask, "Can you help me move the furniture?"

I would say, "Look, I'd love to, but I can't."

And then, of course, you find yourself explaining. When you've got a disease like I did, you walk down the street and no one knows you've got it. If you've got a broken leg, you're on crutches. People get out of the way. But for me, it was not visible. It's not seen. It's a disease of touch. If you would touch me, shake my hand too much, if my belt was too tight, if I sat on a plane seat, carrying groceries, holding children, having sex, anything that involved touch or connection or pressure on the body, my immune system confused that pressure as a break of the skin. My body thought that something had broken the seal, and as such, it alerted the immune army to block off that area, as illustrated in the cartoons in the movie. So I had these mixed messages going on in my body. We needed to straighten it out.

Angie: One of the really exciting things that I heard you talk about last night was that you were going to start doing some medical research.

Joe: I'm trying to bring the medical community into what we're doing. I'm a logical guy. I really can't prove it, but I know that what I did on those five months got me off medication and got me well. You can't really prove that, because you could argue that I could have done everything by eating processed food and done nothing, and just, some act of God, five months later I could have gotten off it. It's never proven.

So what we need to do is work out ways to work with scientists, work with medicine, work with doctors, and find out ways that we can put this to the test, get substantial data that then can be independently verified and written about, and then find our way into the annals of literature so that future generations can look back and say, "You know what? Back in that time 150 years ago, in 2015, there was this group of crazy people around the world that called themselves rebooters. They did all these tests. They did this under supervised conditions at major universities around the world, and this is what they found."

And maybe we'll discover something really cool, or maybe we'll discover something that we don't really understand. But we're going to give it a crack. I think that there's a huge opportunity out in the world for this sort of Mother Nature orientated solution, as opposed to people in white coats trying to solve the problems made by people in white coats.

Shane: Joe, last year you offered a program called Camp Reboot, which I was very fortunate to attend for five days. Can you describe what Camp Reboot is, and tell us what inspired you to create it?

Joe: Camp Reboot is a group of people who come to Rhinebeck, two hours north of New York City, for five days of just juicing. But if you want to eat, we also have little programs on the side, but most people decide to do the juicing only. You get into a small subgroup of 20 people with a health coach and a trainer and a certified nutritionist to monitor. We've got doctors and their tests and labs.

It's really to sort of bring people together, and to enable people to juice with a whole group of people, in this case about 200. This year we're hoping for 500 people. It's an incredible week. We put on courses and workshops. I'm there and we do lots of fun stuff. There's yoga. There's exercise. There are early nights. If you want to get massage treatments you can, but that's extra, of course. But the Omega Institute offers all of that, and the people are fabulous to work with.

It's really a week of inspiration, of education, and of entertainment. It's a little bit like a movie that goes for five days. So, for me, I love it and get a lot out of it. I don't think there was a person that went there last year who didn't leave healthier or happier, and that's saying something. I didn't do the juice only for these five days this year—I just ate plants while I was there. But I know what it's like when you go away and you leave your world, and you go and juice for five days for the first time and you go back home.

So you've only really had a five- or six-day holiday, depending on the travel, but you actually feel like you had a month off. That's really valuable in today's world, where you can get a week's break, but you feel so good that you feel like you've had a month off. When you juice for five days, it feels like a month. So you actually get the best of both worlds.

Shane: As I said, I attended Camp Reboot. I consider myself an experienced juicer, and I left learning a lot. I actually felt much healthier. I made great connections there with people I'm still talking with.

You mentioned there is a program where you can eat at Camp Reboot. My favorite story of those five days was David. His wife was also there. I got talking to them both. David had a fair amount of weight to lose and his wife was very trim, and she said, "I'm going to juice all day and go to the cafeteria in the evening."

I saw them on day three. I said, "How is it going?"

He said, "My wife is doing the whole juice only."

So she juiced the whole way with him.

Angie: Incredible.

Shane: It's so great to have that support from partners and friends, and David went on to lose 50 pounds. Remarkable.

Joe: Well, it's a great way for someone to get started. If you're at home and you failed and you struggled, this is a fabulous kickstart for the five days. I know that not everyone can afford it, and I wish there was some way we could make it cheaper. But it's difficult to put all of this together with the resort infrastructure and have that at our disposal without having this cost.

Angie: It's a lot cheaper than a 30-day vacation, though.

Joe: No, you're not wrong there. It's a lot cheaper. And you're going to save money in the long run with your health too, by the way. But it's a great way to start. If you are beginning, you can use Camp Reboot as the first five days of your journey. Or maybe you are on day seven or eight and struggling. This is a great boost to get you to day 13. And then get you through into what I call an area where you start to experience "Human 2.0"; where you get to feel what it's like to really be a human.

In all honesty, if you've never done three or four days of just juice, then you really haven't experienced what it's like to be a human. You don't know what all of your ancestors, what all of your relatives have been through. Because we come from this history of feast and famine where there wasn't always food around.

So just to experience what it's like to be human, just to sort of have what I call a little travel trip to go from the valley to the top of the mountain, you'll love the view, and you will be excited by the altitude that you've achieved. And when you go back to eating food, if you start eating from what I call the "fun part of town," which is the processed food and the animal products, if you eat too much of that and not enough of the "essential part of town," which is the plant food, then your altitude will start to drop. You won't have as much visibility. The little human inside, who we started this conversation talking about, will come out and say, "You know what? Get back on the plants. You'll want to do that." And you will. You will have some support and assistance from Mother Nature.

Shane: Joe, you are an extremely busy man, and Angie and I, and all the listeners at Juicing Radio, are very grateful that you have given us your time for this interview.

Joe: It's great to be here. What you are doing is awesome. It's so exciting to see what you're doing here. This can lead to millions of people watching and listening to what you are doing and following you. So it's just great to see. It's awesome. I'm seeing so much of this sort of commerce and business and inspiration and excitement that's happening around juicing and around people eating, blending, or drinking more fruits and vegetables. So the future is good.

Shane: Thank you, Joe.

Joe: Thanks, guys.

Angie: Thank you.

Joe: Juice on!

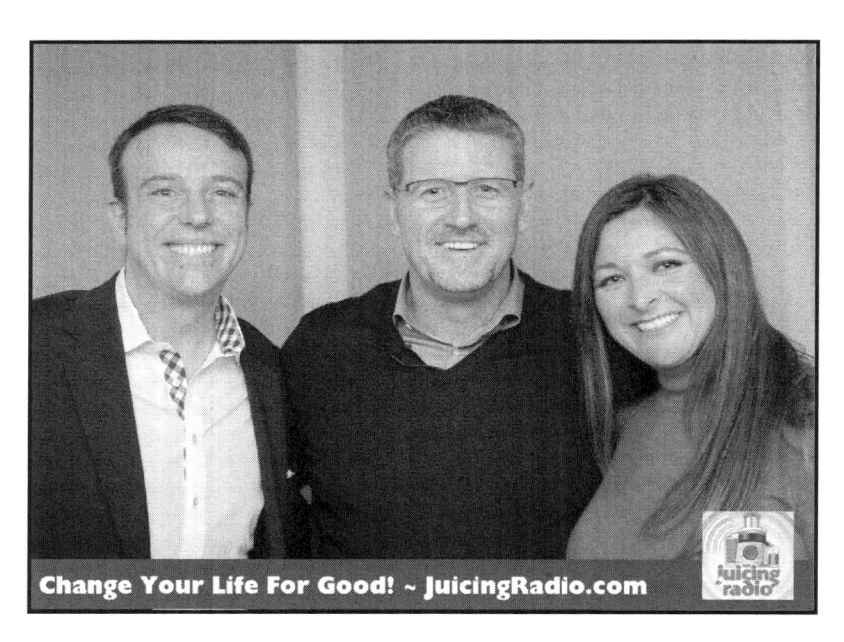

Shane: Wow. That was a great interview with Joe. Wasn't it, Angie?

Angie: It was amazing. It was such a privilege to have Joe answering our listener's questions. It was really something special.

Shane: It was a good interview all around, but what stuck out for you?

Angie: Well, one of the things that stuck out for me was when Joe talked about being perfect. I think a lot of us get caught up in doing things the right way, and I think it can stop us from doing anything at all. He talks about when he goes off into the fun part of town and has a burger or enjoys himself, and his strategy for getting back on track. So he's absolutely not perfect, and I think that kind of gives other people permission to not be perfect either, and not be too hard on themselves.

Shane: Yeah. I think you're right. He's refreshingly honest in his book. He talks about his love of chocolate ice cream, and he has to regulate that. I really enjoyed his answers about alcohol, because it's something I struggle with when I'm trying to be healthy and I go out with the boys to watch football. You go to a bar, you don't go for a beer, but then, what else is there to drink? You don't want to drink Coca-Cola, like Joe was saying. I really liked him talking about those strategies. They are things

I've not really heard him talk about in the past, and when we talked about his grandfather . . .

Angie: That was really moving that he was willing to share that. It's an intimate part of his history. I think it was a special interview. I also enjoyed hearing more about his medical research. That's exciting. It seems like that is, maybe, part three of the reboot with Joe journey. How you move a society forward, right? We have this grassroots effort. People are changing their lives. We have all these great stories, but backing it up with empirical evidence is groundbreaking. It could really change the health of millions of Americans and even people around the world.

Shane: Angie, you were on the TV commercial for *Fat, Sick and Nearly Dead* that was aired on US television. You were also a success story in Joe's book. You've worked with him closer than I have, but I was extremely nervous before this interview. But Joe is a great guy. He's very down to earth. But he has gone out of his way to make a movie, and, as we heard him say, it wasn't for it to be a blockbuster.

Joe has changed so many lives. He has spent so much of his own money on this. This is a legend.

Angie: It was quite an experience. I think the other thing that's really great is that when we asked the questions, he addressed them by name. He's such a down-to-earth guy. I think a lot of people think of him as a legend, but he's one guy who shared his experience with turning his life around, and it has touched millions of people.

Shane: And even calling Joe a legend—I imagine him squirming. That's not what he's about, and I think that's the secret of his success. He's not one of these celebrity TV guys, running along the beach with six-pack abs. Like you said about not being perfect, I don't think he likes to be thought of as a legend, but we certainly think of him as a legend.

If you have been moved by Joe's story, if you've lost weight, if you've fought off a particular health condition, you should buy a copy of his book. I think it's important that Joe sees that people are prepared to put their hands in their pocket and actually support his word. And it's a really good book.

Angie: It is, and it's a really comprehensive book. Out of the hundreds of questions that we got, most of the answers are covered in the book. It's a short read, but it's completely comprehensive, and it includes everything you need to know to get started.

Joe is also very generous. He offers so much free content and help on Reboot with Joe. He also has guided reboots for people who need more support. If you want to go to Camp Reboot, that's another support that he offers. Shane went last year.

Shane: I did. And let me touch on the costs and the investment and what he's doing. He talked about this in the interview, that he made the movie, and then he realized after some time that it was catching on. So he built a comprehensive website where you can get all sorts of information and the meal plans. There's a community on there, and Angie and I are both Reboot ambassadors. I know, for a fact, that the program is not cheap. There's a lot of investment that Joe is making. We've got to be grateful for that.

You mentioned Camp Reboot, and I went last year. What really surprised me was the fact that Joe was around all day, every day. I kind of thought he might turn up for a few hours in the morning, shake a few hands and then disappear. He was around the whole day, every day, and in the evenings. I don't know how he had his energy, to be quite frank. He had time for everybody.

If you're interested in more details about any of the programs, books, or movies we've discussed, please check the Juicing Radio website, or the Resource section of this book.

Get your free copy of
How to Get Started with Juicing
and receive free email juice coaching
(but not spam—that's not healthy).

Sign up at www.juicinghabits.com

JUICING RADIO

Shane and Angie invite you to listen to a juicing success story every week on Juicing Radio.
Sign up for updates and never miss an episode at JuicingRadio.com.

A Must Listen

by EmilyDinWY

I love that Shane and Angie share their own personal success stories. The interviews are great and emphasize that each person's journey to health is different and individual. Anyone can start juicing fruits and veggies, no matter what diet you follow, what your income is, or what your schedule is like. Try 1 juice a day.

Resources

Essential Juicing Websites

Juicing Radio
www.juicingradio.com

Reboot With Joe Cross
www.rebootwithjoe.com

Jay Kordich
www.jaykordich.com

Juicemaster – Jason Vale
www.juicemaster.com

WellnessGuides
www.wellnessguides.org

Natural Juice Junkie
www.naturaljuicejunkie.com

Reboot Phil
www.juicewithphil.com

All About Juicing
http://www.all-about-juicing.com/

ExploreRaw
www.exploreraw.com

HoldingHerOwn
www.holdingherown.com

Prolific Juicing
www.prolificjuicing.com

Kris Carr
www.kriscarr.com

Essential Juicing Movies and Food Documentaries

You can find most of the movies listed below for purchase on DVD on download at

http://juicingradio.com/juicing-movies/

Fat Sick and Nearly Dead
www.fatsickandnearlydead.com

Super Juice Me
www.superjuiceme.com

Food Matters
http://www.foodmatters.tv/

Hungry For Change
http://www.hungryforchange.tv/

Forks Over Knives
http://www.forksoverknives.com/

Powered by Green Smoothies
http://www.fmtv.com/watch/powered-by-green-smoothies

Essential Reading

These are books we have personally read and recommend for anyone who wants to achieve success with their juicing and lifestyle goals. They are on our own bookshelves. We will update the Juicing Book Club page with new juicing related books.

www.juicingbookclub.com

Reboot With Joe Cross Juice Diet – Joe Cross

Reboot With Joe Cross Juice Diet Cook Book – Joe Cross

7 pounds in 7 days Super Juice Diet – Jason Vale
    (the book that got Shane through his first 7 day juice fast!)

Turbo Charge Your Life in 14 Days – Jason Vale

The Big Book of Juices – Natalie Savona

The Best Green Drinks Ever – Katrine Van Wyk

The Healthy Juicers Bible – Farnoosh Brock

Once I Was Fat – Zach Bohanon

Juicing for Athletes – Brian Pace

The Miracle Juice Diet – Amanda Cross

The Juiceman's Power of Juicing – Jay Kordich

The Complete Idiots Guide to Juice Fasting – Steve Prussack

Green for Life – Victoria Boutenko

Sexy Crazy Cancer – Kris Carr

Main Street Vegan – Victoria Moran

Awaken the Giant Within – Anthony Robbins

Goals! – Brian Tracy

End of Dieting – Dr Joel Fuhrman

A Course in Weight Loss – Marianne Williamson

About the Authors

Angela von Buelow, born in Texas and raised in California, is a former foodie. In fact, Angie once ran a popular restaurant review site in San Francisco.

Angie achieved 86 pounds of weight loss through juicing and has completed two half marathons. (Both Angie and Shane could not run for 1 minute before juicing.)

Angie has appeared on *The Dr. Oz Show* talking about her juicing success. She was a featured success story in *The Reboot with Joe Juice Diet: Lose Weight, Get Healthy, and Feel Amazing.*

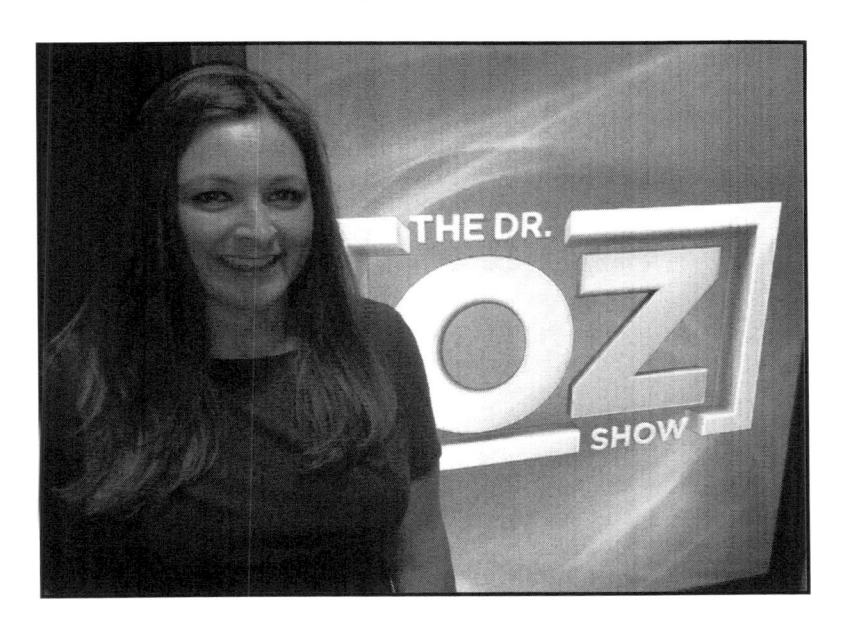

Shane Whaley started juicing in 2010 (after several failed attempts.) Shane has lost 80 pounds (6 stone) and has completed four half marathons. He set up the Running On Juice blog, which he started in early 2010 when he began his amazing journey and juicing weight loss. He wrote a Free Juicing Starter Guide in 2011, which has been downloaded more than 25,000 times.

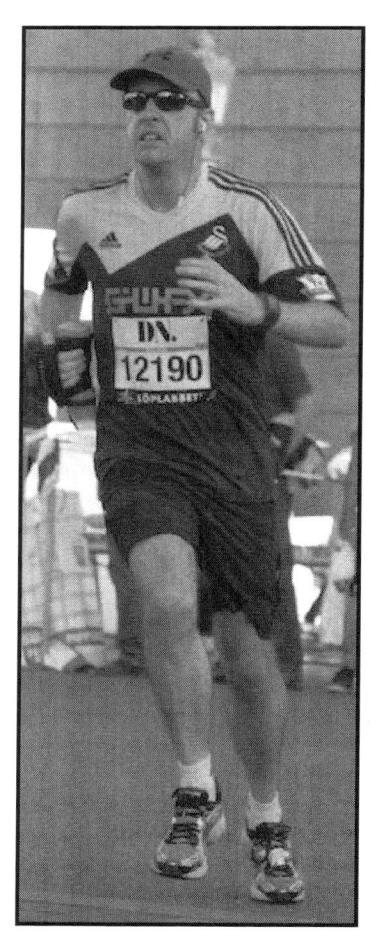

Shane started the Juicing Radio podcast when he realized that a weekly podcast with free juicing content would have helped him in his early days.

In November 2013, with Angela von Buelow, he launched JuicingRadio.com, a weekly juicing podcast, which is listened to by thousands of people every week.

Shane is a Brit who lived in Stockholm, Sweden, before moving to San Francisco and later New York City, where he lives with his greyhound, Brunhilde. He loves soccer, reading, and Morrissey!

Connect with Social Media

JUICING RADIO

http://www.juicingradio.com

FACEBOOK

http://www.facebook.com/juicingradio

TWITTER

http://twitter.com/juicingradio

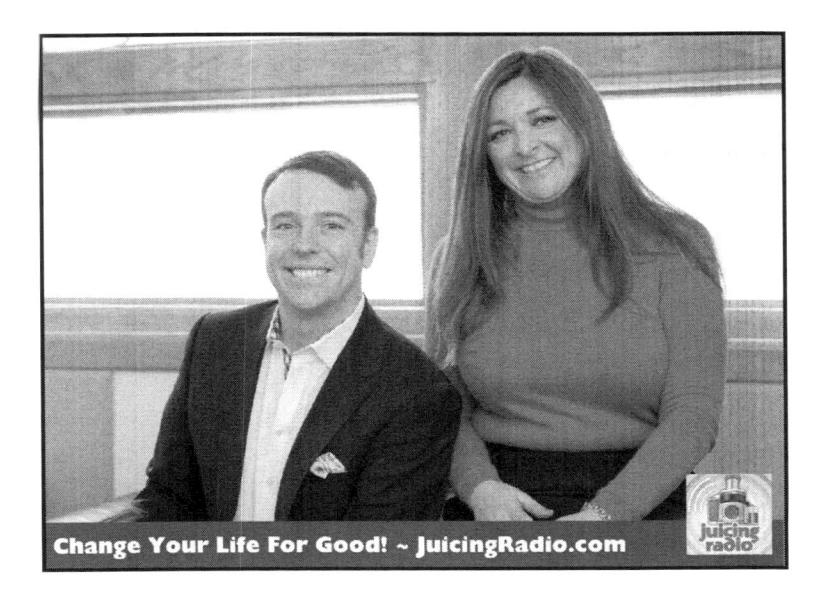

Made in the USA
San Bernardino, CA
16 December 2014